The Foundations Of Nutrition

First published in 2024
by Leeds & London Partnership

15-17 High March, Daventry,
Northants NN11 4HB, UK

A CIP catalogue record of this book is
available from the British Library

ISBN 978-1-7391378-1-6

The information in this book is
designed to be advisory and helpful.
It is not intended to treat or diagnose
any medical conditions and is not a
substitute for professional medical
advice. Please consult your GP before
starting, changing or stopping any
medical treatment. The author and
publisher are not responsible for any
liability arising directly or indirectly
from the use or misuse of the
information contained in this book.

Foreword

Foreword by **Phil Beard BSc (Hons), MSc,**
Nutritionist and Nutrition Trainer

My journey to nutrition started working in the NHS as a dietician and all too often I saw the negative impacts a poor diet can have on our lives. Food is what nourishes us but the demand for convenience and speed have taken priority. We eat on-the-go more than ever, ultra processed food (UPF) is everywhere and it's hard to avoid it. So much so that around 25-60% of daily energy intake comes from these foods. This varies from country to country but in the UK the figure is over 50%. The trouble is an ultra-processed food is hard to spot, especially when so many daily staples fall into this category.

Officially, UPF's are ready-to-eat industrially formulated products that are made mostly or entirely from substances derived from foods and additives. Simply put, this is anything with ingredients you would not find in your kitchen at home. Examples include packaged baked goods (especially bread) and snacks, fizzy drinks, cereals, ready meals, dehydrated vegetable soups, reconstituted meat and fish products and many plant based alternatives. On top of the usual chemicals they contain for flavouring, colouring, stabilising, emulsifying and preserving, they often contain high levels of added sugar, fat and salt and they are lacking in vitamins and fibre.

Eating these foods occasionally is ok but research shows regular consumption can have a significant negative effect. One study of 105,159 French adults showed consumption of ultra-processed food in the diet was associated with significantly higher rates of overall cardiovascular disease, coronary heart disease, and cerebrovascular disease. A second study of 19,899 Spanish adults showed that higher consumption of ultra-processed foods (more than 4 servings per day) was associated with a 62% increased risk of all cause mortality. For each additional daily serving of ultra-processed food, mortality risk increased by 18%.

These are dauting figures but there are things we can do and the good news is this book will help you with some simple steps to get your foundations right. Use it is a guide to help you reach optimum nutrient levels, achieve good digestive health and attain a greater feeling of wellbeing. I've seen many people successfully improve their diet and feel better, you can do the same.

It can be good fun trying new foods and recipes so enjoy this time of discovery and remember, always check the ingredient lists of the foods you buy and ask yourself, is this ingredient there to help me or to help the manufacturer. If it's the latter, leave it on the shelf.

Phil Beard

BSc (Hons) MSc

Introduction

The world of nutrition can be a confusing place, how do we truly know if we are eating the correct variety of foods to provide all the nutrients necessary for health?

We all feel a bit under the weather or not quite 100% some days and that's our body's way of telling us that we are lacking in something. We often push ourselves through these times but what if there was a way to be abundantly healthy, to have balanced energy and achieve ongoing wellness?

This book will take you through how nutrition can give you the energy, focus and zest you need. By the end of this guide, you'll have a clear understanding of the fundamental choices required for health - in food, lifestyle and supplementation. The Foundations of Nutrition are clarified in three steps: optimum intake, gut health and inflammation.

We will explore how nutrient deficiency and nutrient optimisation can be addressed with diet, personalised multivitamins and minerals, how gut health can be improved through targeted probiotics and take a deep dive into how fish oils and plant-based nutritional oils reduce inflammation. This triple-barrelled approach will simplify, yet maximise the impact of your health regimen.

Make the Foundations of Nutrition part of your daily routine to create new habits of a lifetime.

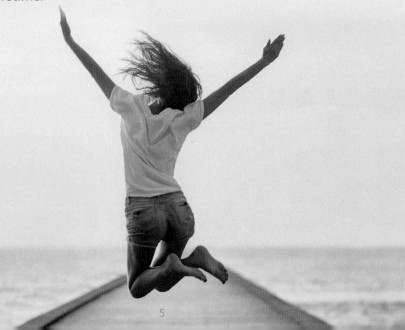

The Journey to Abundant Health

Abundant health is not just the absence of pain, or the occasional decent night's sleep, it is about positive energy, strength and uplifted mood. With the right dietary and lifestyle choices, you can fuel your body to a greater level of nutrient density that will make you healthier, happier and better able to live the life you want.

In this book we will cover:

- **What we eat, why it matters and the potential repercussions.**
  You will learn how to tell if you are deficient in certain nutrients, what the signs and symptoms are, and the reasons that nutrient status can become too low. We will explore what a poor nutrient intake means in terms of health and how it can drive inflammation and impair digestive health.

- **Managing health conditions.**
  It is not a secret that a significant proportion of the UK population are managing a health condition and their prevalence is on the rise. We will look at how nutrition is linked to the development of health conditions and how long-term health conditions can lead to the development of further illnesses.

In addition, we will highlight when specific nutrients may be required in larger volumes than the average diet may provide to help manage long term conditions.

- **Why food is becoming less nutritious.**
  The history of nutrition is an interesting story of how we learnt from accidental malnourishment to reveal the role of each known nutrient in the body. We'll look at how these learning points shape the application of nutrition to daily life, and we will also look at the importance of lifestyle. Food history includes the agricultural revolution which started in the late 17th century, whereby a greater demand was placed on agriculture which led to the development of intensive farming. This has created a domino effect, reducing the nutrient density of vegetables, fruits and other produce and ultimately conferring the lowered nutrient density to those who consume the produce. A combination of both the agricultural and industrial revolution produced a new and current way of eating, which is referred to as the Western diet.

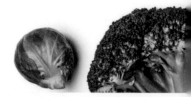

- **The rise of convenience.**
  A shift in our lifestyle has occurred, whereby we spend much less time than our ancestors in preparing and eating food, consequently we eat on-the-go more than ever. We'll review why the need for speed means we often compromise our diet and share some solutions on how to manage this.

- **The impact of medication on diet.**
  Medical interventions and medications have been life savers; however, they have an impact on what we need to eat to utilise them within the body. We will investigate what you need to know about nutrition and medication.

- **The nutrient trinity.**
  Learn about micronutrients, nutritional oils and beneficial bacteria. Micronutrients are the vitamins and minerals our bodies need to function and we'll go through essential fatty acids, what they are and how much you need. Beneficial bacteria are our miniscule friends, we will look at the benefits they confer and easy ways to include them in the diet.

- **Which vitamins and minerals.**
  The necessary intake of vitamins and minerals can vary dependant on lifestyle, age, and health status. Each life phase will be discussed, and advice and tips provided to optimise nutritional intake. In addition, at various stages in life, certain health conditions or health goals may be apparent, for example, fertility and reproductive health, while alongside menopause the risk of cardiovascular outcomes or osteoporosis may increase.

- **Support.**
  And finally, we'll show you where to seek further advice and information.

This is going to be an in depth and enlightening read, so settle in with your favourite herbal tea and let's get started.

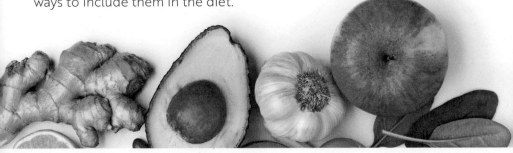

Why Diet Matters

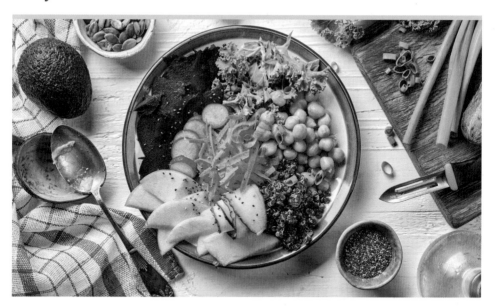

It is common to hear the phrase "you are what you eat" and that's because diet, along with lifestyle has been largely associated with health, or lack thereof, throughout every stage of life from developing babies to the elderly.

But why is this?

Nutrition is the consumption of compounds known as nutrients in the form of food. Nutrients are classified as large and small (macro and micro) in reference to their molecular size. Macronutrients, are carbohydrates, fats, protein, and fibre that make up a large proportion of wholefoods.

> **The highly calorific Western diet is actually considered close to malnourishment**

Micronutrients consist of vitamins, minerals, and trace elements, in addition to plant specific nutrients known as phytonutrients. Micronutrients, in turn, account for a small but dense proportion of wholefoods.

You'll note the mention of wholefoods and this refers to foods that are entire and have not undergone any form of processing. They are essentially as close to their natural state as possible. Wholefoods are extremely nutrient dense. Ideally, 80% of what we eat should be wholefoods.
By eating in this manner, it will naturally reduce our intake of processed foods.
However, if you are unsure, a good test for processed foods is to check the ingredients list.

If you read items that you've never heard of and are difficult to pronounce, it is likely the food is highly processed.

The reason nutrients are so important is because the human body is a continuous series of molecular transformations that require specific nutrients to function. In the case of magnesium or zinc, for example, both nutrients are known to be involved in over 300 enzymatic processes, which include blood pressure regulation, taste, energy and sleep.

> ## 66 80% of our diet should be made up of wholefoods 99

Diet is so important that long-term nutrient insufficiencies can contribute to the development of chronic health conditions such as osteoporosis. Even short term insufficient nutrient intake impacts body processes, for example, sleep quality may deteriorate, or stress becomes difficult to manage. Eating a healthy diet may be difficult for some people who live hectic lifestyles, work long hours, or have poor access to healthful foods. Age may affect the nutrients we need and for those who already have a health condition, or multiple conditions and take medication, further nutrient insufficiencies are likely to occur.

Malnourishment - the phenomenon of the Western diet

We are living longer which might suggest we have the right diet. But health conditions that develop because of lifestyle and diet are on the rise, each of which incur a huge healthcare cost. Each year a staggering £8.8 billion is spent to treat cases of Type II Diabetes. By the year 2035, it's estimated that 5 million people in England will have the disease, which can negatively affect vision, kidney health, heart disease and incidence of stroke. One of the leading factors for Type II Diabetes is diet and specifically, the Western diet. Characteristic of this is the consumption of processed foods which are particularly prevalent in developed countries and considered a contributing factor. This way of eating is highly calorific but provides few nutrients, subsequently and perhaps shockingly, it is considered close to malnourishment.

The Western diet is a nutritional phenomenon. More people carry excess weight than ever before with around 60% of the population now overweight or obese.

Carrying excess weight can be obviously visible but may also be hidden. Visceral fat is fat that wraps around your abdominal organs. You can't always feel it or see it. For example you could have a flat stomach and still have visceral fat.

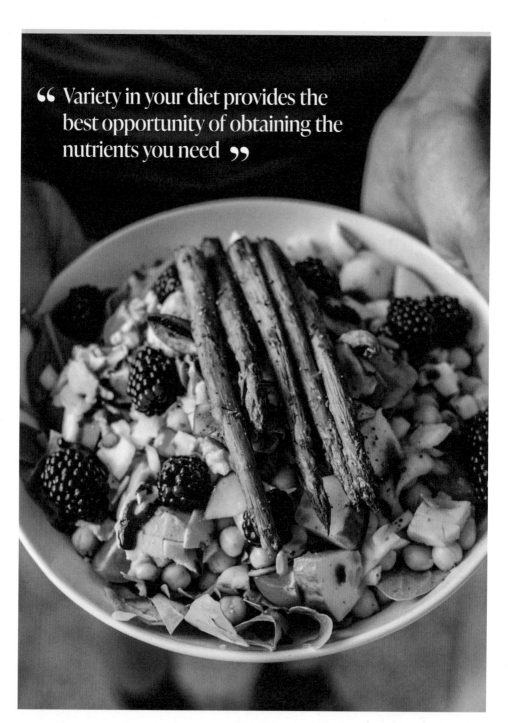

> **"** Variety in your diet provides the best opportunity of obtaining the nutrients you need **"**

Being overweight has implications for health on its own. This state of excessive caloric intake with low nutrient provision not only brings about elevated body mass, but also a malnourished state where key nutrients are missing. The Western diet is considered a result of an amalgamation of the need for high food production (i.e. more mouths to feed) and technological advances. This was thought to be the answer to a growing, time-strapped population to provide quick and easy meal solutions such as fast foods, processed ready meals and sauces that have replaced traditional food preparation. The problem lies in that these foods use large amounts of salt as a preservative and taste enhancer, low nutrient ingredients and alternating layers of fats and sugar to create a nice mouth feel and desire. Thus, large amounts of sodium, trans fats and sugar are consumed at the loss of vitamins, minerals and trace elements that are necessary for health. Furthermore despite being highly calorific they don't satisfy the appetite very well so you are likely to eat more.

> ❝ Those who think they have no time for healthy eating, will sooner or later have to find time for illness ❞
> – Edward Stanley

With so many time pressures and demands, many of us are eating foods characteristic of a Western diet. For example, simple carbohydrate foods that elevate blood glucose, such as ready meals, sweets, cakes, and white bread, as well as highly processed meats, which are high in hydrogenated fats, salt, and additives such as preservatives, binders, and colourants. It also includes pre-prepared sauces and processed ingredients such as spreads, some cheeses, chips and even sometimes ready-to-cook vegetables.

> ❝ Diet is associated with health through every life stage ❞

Over time, an inadequate intake of nutrients can drive a suboptimal status in organ and tissue function. For example, long term stress, exercise, and pollution damage cells within the body. A suboptimal supply of nutrients reduces the ability to repair those cells which in turn makes tissues less resistant to infections and illnesses. Our bodies are amazing and sophisticated biological structures, whereby every function relies on an adequate intake of good quality nutrients. Wholefoods that are naturally brightly coloured indicates significant nutrient density and so the aim is to consume a variety of different coloured foods to supply a host of high quality nutrition.

Eating for Health

So what is the right diet?

With such a vast array of food choices, it is easy to choose foods based on taste rather than the nutrients supplied. Nutrition is essential for growth and development plus health and wellbeing. Eating a healthy diet can be protective of future illnesses and improve your quality of life.

> 66 Don't eat anything your great-great grandparents wouldn't recognize as food. In fact there are a great many food-like items in the supermarket your ancestors wouldn't recognize 99
> – Michael Pollan

The message in Michael Pollan's quote is powerful, and it emphasises that foods which are unprocessed and brightly coloured are the richest in nutrition. A traditional style of eating which demonstrates the truth of the quote is the classic Mediterranean diet which comprises of vegetables, salad items, olives, legumes, wholegrains and nuts and seeds, plus a few servings of fish, poultry, eggs or meat weekly.
By filling the diet with natural foods, processed and sugar laden foods such as ready meals, pizza, pasta, cakes, sweets and pastries are naturally eliminated.

The traditional Mediterranean diet can be considered a wholefoods diet as the food items are fresh from the surrounding area and simply prepared. The Mediterranean lifestyle also encourages working outdoors, growing and raising your own food and social connection in the community.

Variety is the key to a good diet and a good starting place is to eat wholefoods. Aim for at least one serving of each colour of the rainbow daily. For example vegetables, salad items and fruit and add to this a source of protein. Also include wholegrains or potatoes and finally a sprinkling of seeds, nuts, or a plant oil. If you are buying prepared foods, check the ingredients list to see if there are additives or preservatives. If there are unusual names and things you haven't heard of, it is likely to be a processed food.

After a few weeks consider your diet for opportunities to tweak and alter food choices to improve total nutrient intake and variety. It's great to keep a diary that you can refer back to.

Whilst following the above guide is ideal, it is still hard to know if you're getting all the nutrients you need from your diet.

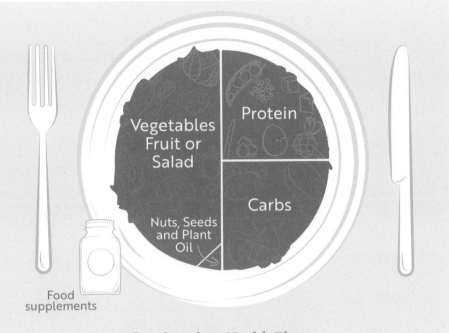

The Abundant Health Plate

Aim to incorporate different food groups into every meal

½ vegetables, salad and fruit · ¼ protein · ¼ carbohydrate
Plus some nuts, seeds and plant oil

There are some indicators you can look out for. Classic signs that your nutrient intake may be suboptimal include prolonged tiredness, difficulty in recovering from exercise, an increase in stress and a decline in sleep quality, besides frequent infections, poor skin condition or lowered mood. It can be easy to fall into using quick fixes, foods that are pre-prepared rather than cooked, like ready meals, fast food or chocolate.

The Rainbow Challenge

To see whether you're already eating a truly 'rainbow' diet, write down every food you eat for a week in a list form – ie: tomatoes, cheese, cauliflower etc – have you eaten more than 25 different items in 7 days?

Low temperature cooking and steaming using wholefoods is the best way to maximise nutrients and minimise processed foods. Wholefoods will provide complex carbohydrates and fats as an energy source, which are slow releasing and will provide a balanced supply of energy so that you are less likely to opt for a quick sugar fix.
It does take more time but preparing in advance and batch booking can help.

Consider when in the week is the best time to prepare healthy meals, so that on busy days you have a meal in the freezer and do not opt for a processed choice. Supporting your diet with supplementation may also help provide optimal nutritional status.

Signs you may be nutrient deficient

Infections	Sleep issues	Poor digestion
Increase in stress	Slower brain function	Low mood
Lethargy	Reduced recovery	Poor skin condition

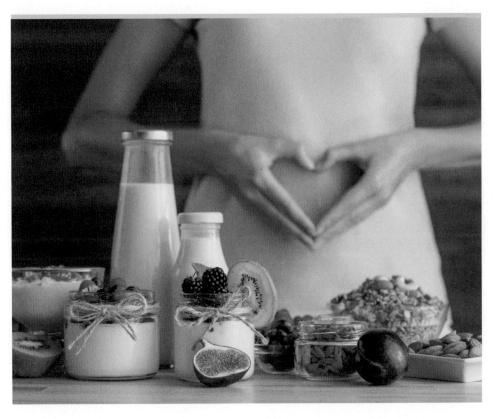

We've touched on how nutrients are important for the body to work at optimum levels and now we'll look in more detail at why.

The digestive tract – the first line of defence

The digestive tract, commonly referred to as the gut, incorporates the mouth, oesophagus, stomach, pancreas, and gallbladder followed by the small and large intestine and bowel.
Maintaining a healthy digestive system is crucial because the whole tract is a complex interplay of tissues, organs and signalling receptors that work in harmony to digest food and release nutrients for absorption into the blood supply. Think of it like the processing plant to extract the compounds your body needs to work effectively. Any block in the process will reduce the efficiency and leave you feeling low on energy or not quite 100%.

Additionally, the digestive tract is the first line of defence against bacteria, virus, fungi and foreign agents, subsequently when this organ is not functioning correctly the body is at greater risk of an infection.

The Link to Inflammation

Food intolerance can be caused by a number of things including genetic predisposition, abnormal immune response or contamination.

The root of food intolerances

Eating a Western diet, made up of processed foods, over a prolonged period can be a contributing factor to developing an impaired gut and food intolerances such as gluten, dairy or caffeine, which can be associated with impaired digestive tract function. It is considered that the cells that line the digestive tract may allow undigested particles of food to slip through into circulation when in a state of stress or infection. When immune cells detect the food particles, they create an immune response, as though they are infectious bacteria or a foreign agent. This results in the body displaying symptoms like bloating, rashes and headaches amongst others. Our bodies have a clever memory function which means each time that food is consumed, the immune system recognises it as a threat and reacts accordingly.

Useful as this memory function may be for identifying true hazardous compounds, it isn't helpful for food and may mean certain foods have to be eliminated from the diet to avoid symptoms that can cause significant discomfort. Not only it is uncomfortable, immune activation is also a nutrient hungry operation.

The body's number one goal is the preservation of life, and so this will influence how nutrients are used within the body.

If there is a perceived deficit or damage to tissues, then specific nutrients will be directed to support the repair of those tissues. However, when the body is low on important nutrients, these tissues will not be correctly fuelled, repaired, or protected and ultimately will result in poor or even impaired function. This, along with stress, pollution, food additives such as emulsifiers, as well as bacteria or viruses cause an inflammatory environment.

The mystery of inflammation

Although the word inflammation brings to mind images of swelling, heat and pain, and this would be true of inflammation associated with a visible injury, inflammation can be largely invisible and undetected.

Inflammation is the first stage of the immune response; it aims to neutralise a foreign or infective agent through heat and fluid, which then triggers healing. Therefore, inflammation is common, however there is a variation in the duration of the inflammatory response, subsequently, efficient inflammation is short lived whereas long term inflammation is associated with long term health conditions.

At this point it should be highlighted that short-term inflammation is good. It is a sign of a healthy immune system, it protects the body from infection and triggers healing. However, when inflammation becomes chronic, which is defined as long term that lasts from several months to years, it is a health problem.

> **❝ Inflammation can be largely invisible and undetected ❞**

Common signs and symptoms of long-term inflammation are body pain, fatigue and low mood, besides digestive issues such as constipation, diarrhoea and acid reflux, plus changes in body weight and frequent infections. In the modern world, the body is exposed to pollution, additives, excipients, and toxins that each contribute to stimulating the immune system which then further generates inflammation.

Common signs of long-term inflammation

Body Pain	Fatigue	Low Mood
Constipation	Diarrhoea	Acid Reflux
Frequent Infections	Skin Conditions	Changes in Body weight

This puts an even greater demand on nutrient provision from the diet which if compromised to start with, will mean immune supporting nutrients may become suboptimal, and the inflammation perpetuates.

Research has identified common risk factors that promote a long-lasting inflammatory state:

- **Age**
  Increasing age is associated with an increase in certain signalling agents that incite inflammation.
- **Obesity**
  Fat tissue can produce hormones and so secretes inflammatory signalling agents. Subsequently, research shows that body mass index is proportionally related to inflammation.
- **Diet**
  Foods rich in saturated fats, trans fats or refined sugar is associated with greater inflammation.
- **Smoking**
  Smoking is associated with a lower volume of anti-inflammatory signalling agents that would normally regulate inflammation.
- **Stress and poor sleep**
  Both physical and psychological stress are inflammatory. Plus, stress can affect sleep which too drives inflammation.

Managing these areas and working to ensure you have a wholefoods-based diet with optimal nutrients will help to minimise long-term inflammation and the risk of chronic inflammatory diseases.

Shockingly, chronic inflammatory diseases are the most significant cause of death worldwide. In fact, the World Health Organisation considers such diseases as the greatest threat to human health. This is demonstrated by the fact that three out of five people worldwide die due to chronic inflammatory diseases such as, stroke, respiratory diseases, heart disorders, obesity and diabetes.

The malnourishment, digestive health and inflammatory connection

A state of malnutrition, poor digestive health and inflammation drive a perpetuating cycle of health deterioration. This connection is at the root of the increase in non-communicable diseases or NCDs as they are known.

These are conditions that cannot be passed from person to person but develop dependant on their physiological state, such as, Type II Diabetes, cardiovascular diseases, metabolic syndrome and obesity. Subsequently this state of illness may promote the development of concurrent illnesses, a topic we will look at in the next section.

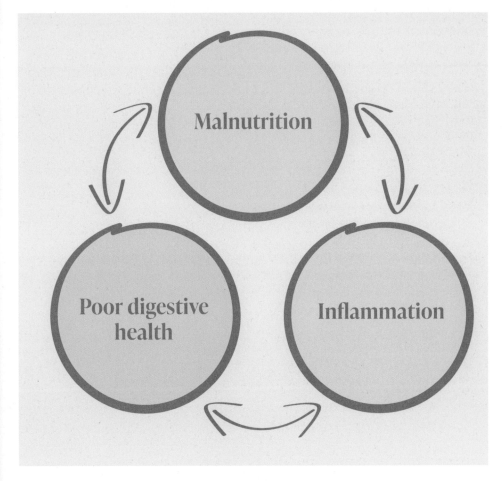

Long Term Health Conditions

Avoiding long-term inflammation and the risk of developing a chronic health condition is what we would all like to achieve. However over 15 million people in the UK live with one long-term health condition, and around three million have three or more. This has a huge impact on quality of life, families, communities, and healthcare. Three or more long term health conditions are generally more common in those over the age of 65 years; however, a trend has begun that shows people under the age of 65 years developing additional health conditions.

Coronary heart disease closely followed by diabetes and depression are the most common long-term health conditions. There is a clear link between long-term health conditions and diet. For example, Type II Diabetes Mellitus is the inability to efficiently manage blood glucose. In normal health, insulin is secreted in response to a spike in blood glucose, such as that after a meal. However, in diabetes, the insulin secretion is delayed, or insufficient and the glucose remains elevated which can cause tissue damage.

Subsequently, foods that are rich in simple carbohydrates, such as sugar, sugar derivatives, white bread, white rice, cakes and pastries cause a greater glucose spike and therefore require efficient insulin secretion. In the case of Type II Diabetes this does not occur and so the glucose crystalises in the blood and may damage the tissues of the blood vessels, kidneys, nerves and eyes. This demonstrates how one long term health condition can promote the development of further health conditions.

> We're living through major health pandemics of obesity, heart disease and depression, all of which are influenced by diet and nutrition.

66 Over 15 million people in the UK live with one long-term health condition 99

20

Long term health concerns can lead to multiple conditions

1st condition	2nd condition	3rd condition
Coronary heart disease	Diabetes	Chronic kidney disease
Diabetes	Coronary heart disease	Chronic kidney disease
Diabetes	Chronic pain	Depression
Diabetes	Chronic pain	Chronic kidney disease
Diabetes	Stroke / TIA	Chronic kidney disease
Diabetes	Chronic kidney disease	Chronic pain
Diabetes	Chronic kidney disease	Chronic heart disease
Diabetes	Depression	Chronic pain
Diabetes	Coronary heart disease	Heart failure
Depression	Morbid obesity	Diabetes

→ Long-term conditions →

Kings College London, (2018). From one to many: Exploring people's progression to multiple long-term conditions in an urban environment. Guy's & St Thomas' Charity. 1 (1), P1-55.

Collateral damage

The symptoms characteristic of long term health conditions can affect other body systems, for example, Type II Diabetes can affect the kidneys, blood vessels, nerves and eyes which can then lead to kidney disease, hardening of the arteries and cardiovascular disease, peripheral neuropathy (nerve damage) or diabetic retinopathy which can cause blindness.

The collateral cascade can be demonstrated in other long term health conditions, for example, Depression is inflammatory, theorised to be a state of inflammation in the brain which may lead to an increase of inflammation in the body. In addition, depression may trigger changes in behaviour, lifestyle and dietary patterns which may lead to a sedentary lifestyle, increase the prevalence of smoking and alcohol consumption, and promote the consumption of simple carbohydrates. Each of these factors can increase the risk of developing Type II Diabetes, obesity or metabolic syndrome.

A Shared pathology

An alternative contributor for the development of further health conditions is that the conditions share the same development pattern. For instance, the generation of inflammation and cellular damage when concentrated in specific tissues promotes the development of disease. For example, we know that Type II Diabetes can damage the blood vessels through elevated blood glucose. The normal response to tissue damage is inflammation and the recruitment of platelets and calcium to form a scab. In the case of continual damage to the blood vessels this becomes a bigger and bigger scab and becomes atherosclerosis which is hardening of the arteries and contributes to cardiovascular disease.

And finally, long-term inflammation may be an indicator that immune activation has become imbalanced which means that inflammation may spread to other tissues and organs in an uncontrolled manner.

The nutrition connection

Let's remain with the Type II Diabetes example. Several B vitamins, zinc and chromium are necessary for the production of insulin and its activity at a cellular level. Therefore, if the individual has suboptimal levels of these nutrients in addition to a simple carbohydrate rich diet, then insulin production, secretion and activity will be compromised. Granted, there can also be genetic, physiological and toxin damage that can contribute, we cannot wholly blame dietary intake, but it certainly plays a contributing factor.

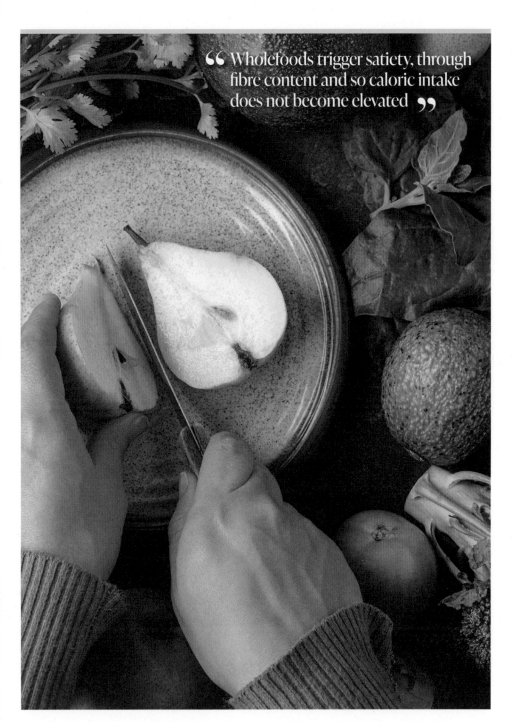

"Wholefoods trigger satiety, through fibre content and so caloric intake does not become elevated"

The Western Diet

An inconvenient truth

The Western diet is built on convenience whether that be enhanced taste, enhanced output or minimal cooking time. An array of meal solutions have been developed to feed a growing population cheaply and conveniently, however, as we have seen in previous chapters, this convenience also provides an inadequate quantity of nutrition to support the modern lifestyle. Its development saw the introduction of food staples, such as grain cereals and processing procedures during the industrial revolution. This changed small scale food production to large scale, single crop monocultures that produce large volumes of food cheaply which fundamentally altered several characteristics of the traditional pre-industrial era diet:

- **Glycaemic load.**
  Namely the amount of carbohydrate per 100 grams of a food. Examples include the selective breeding of wheat and rice for increased output and caloric density.
- **Fatty acid composition.**
  Processing reduces the nutritional value of fats, as demonstrated by refined oils which added a huge calorie intake to the diet. Plus fats are added in food processing which delay satiety and improve taste and mouth feel. Intensively reared animals with an excess of fat tend to be dominant in saturated fat whereas free range animals have a greater proportion of poly- and monounsaturated fat.
- **Macronutrient composition.**
  Grain cereals grown today are vastly different from the traditional diet. Grain cereals are selected for large-scale production based on their high carbohydrate and high fat nutrient profiles, for example, wheat and rapeseed.
- **Micronutrient density.**
  Repeat cropping without a remineralisation programme can lead to mineral deficits in soils. This is further impacted when the crop is refined, it is stripped of its nutritional value.
- **Acid base balance.**
  After digestion, absorption and transformation, most foods release either acid or bicarbonate into circulation, thus influencing an acid or alkaline environment in the body. Acid promoting foods which are more prevalent in the Western diet pressure pH regulation which relies on the consumption of alkaline promoting foods for balance. If alkaline promoting foods are not present then minerals are leached from bone and tooth to maintain pH balance. Acid promoting foods include meats, cereal grains, eggs and cheese, and alkaline promoting foods include vegetables, fruit and salad items.

- **Sodium-potassium ratio.**
  This has been highly affected by the addition of salt to food as a preservative and flavour enhancer. Sodium and potassium play a role in blood pressure and a sodium dominant diet can be associated with increased blood pressure values.
- **Fibre content.**
  The proportion of fibre in the Western diet is far lower than Public Health recommendations. Refined foods, oils, dairy and alcohol are devoid of fibre, and although touted as fibre rich, grains are processed in a manner that reduces their fibre content.

These changes in the nutrient profile of food are considered to play a large role in the development not only of a single health condition but multiple health conditions. This eating pattern is systematically reducing the nutrient density of food that is eaten so that daily living is not fully supported by the necessary nutrient volume. The daily deficit that accumulates may appear incremental but can lead to long term insufficiencies which leave the body open to infection and illnesses.

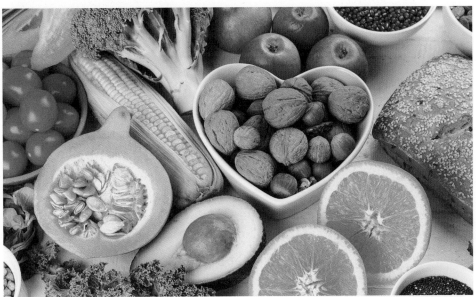

Fibre rich foods include wholegrains, fruit such as berries, pears, melon and oranges, vegetables such as broccoli, carrots and sweetcorn, peas, beans and pulses as well as nuts and seeds.

Nutrient deficiency

Knowing you need certain nutrients is only part of the story. More difficult is understanding if you are deficient and what nutrients you might need more of. There are some common signs which are linked to specific nutrient deficiencies detailed in the table below.

The nutrient deficiency table is not to replace clinical care, a GP should be consulted in the case of new symptom development and if symptoms do not cease.

If you are prescribed medication, please discuss any potential supplementation with your healthcare professional.

Common Symptoms	Potential Dietary Insufficiency
Tiredness and Fatigue	• Complex carbohydrates • B vitamins - especially B3, B5, B6, B12 and folate • Magnesium • Iron • Zinc
Low Mood	• Complete protein • Omega-3 essential fatty acids • B vitamins – especially B1, B2, B3, B5, B6, B12, folate and choline • Magnesium • Zinc • Probiotics / fermented foods
Stress	• B vitamins – especially B5, B6, B12 and folate • Vitamin C • Magnesium • Zinc • Probiotics / fermented foods
High Blood Pressure	• Potassium • Magnesium • Omega-3 essential fatty acids
High Cholesterol	• Vitamin C • Vitamin B3
Hardening Blood Vessels	• Vitamins K2 and D3 • Zinc • Magnesium

Weak Bones	• Calcium • Boron • Magnesium • Vitamin C • Vitamins K2 and D3
Hormonal Imbalance	• Magnesium • Vitamin B6 • Zinc • Omega-3 essential fatty acids
Digestive Health Issues	• Glutamine • Protein • Choline • Probiotics / fermented foods
Sleep Issues	• Protein sources that provide Glycine, Carnitine and Tryptophan • Magnesium • Vitamin C • Complex carbohydrates
Frequent Infections	• Zinc • Selenium • Vitamin C • Vitamin D • Probiotics / fermented foods
Inflammation	• Vitamin D • Vitamin C • Zinc • Selenium • Omega-3 essential fatty acids • Probiotics / fermented foods
Blood Glucose Management	• B vitamins • Zinc • Chromium

Nutrition Isn't New

Although modern research has revealed benefits on the effects of diet, nutrition is not a new phenomenon. The acknowledgement of specific nutrients and their benefit to human health was first realised in the 18th century when upon landing after several months at sea, scurvy-riddled sailors saw a resolution in the characteristic skin and gum lesions. This accidental malnourishment due to the time spent at sea and consuming long life food provisions had depleted their bodies of vitamin C, which resulted in the onset of scurvy.

In 1912, Casimir Funk noted that unprocessed rice protected chickens from a particular illness and coined the term 'vital amine' which was shortened to 'vitamin', and the compound that was present in the rice husk was named vitamin B1, thiamine.

This kickstarted a huge interest in single nutrient research and led to the addition of iodine to table salt, vitamin D fortification of milk and crucially, the first multivitamin and mineral formulation in 1940.

Considered an accident of nutrition history, the demonstration of single nutrient related illnesses led to the fortification of foods or the creation of a public health message. Therefore, nutrients such as iodine and folic acid attracted fortification or an associated public health message respectively. This increased knowledge, associated with nutrients and food, and highlights the chasm between the nutrition that the human body requires versus what is available.

> 66 The word 'diet' is derived from the Greek word 'diaita' meaning 'way of life' 99

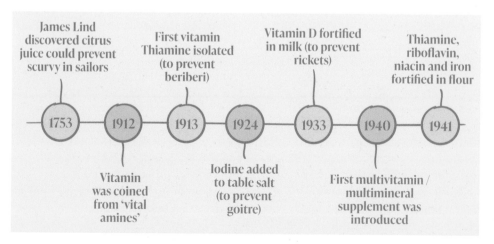

James Lind discovered citrus juice could prevent scurvy in sailors — **1753**

Vitamin was coined from 'vital amines' — **1912**

First vitamin Thiamine isolated (to prevent beriberi) — **1913**

Iodine added to table salt (to prevent goitre) — **1924**

Vitamin D fortified in milk (to prevent rickets) — **1933**

First multivitamin / multimineral supplement was introduced — **1940**

Thiamine, riboflavin, niacin and iron fortified in flour — **1941**

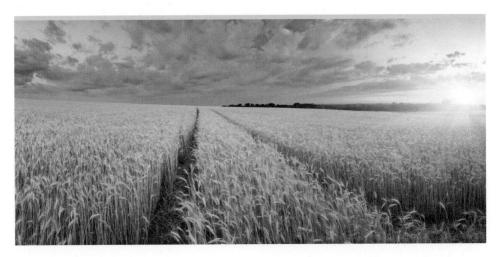

How food production has changed nutrition

In the pre 1800s, subsistence was provided by each family via home garden production. Which, as the century progressed, became pressured by an increase in human survival rate and longevity that tripled the population. Agricultural farming intensified through new systems such as the rotation of fewer crops, more produce per m^2 and land reclamation, for example fens were drained to be used for crops. Crop yields were manipulated by replacing low yielding crops with higher yielding, such as wheat and barley. This was closely followed by fodder crops, so that animals could be kept in sheds to preserve land for crops. At a similar time, it was discovered that the introduction of nitrogen would increase crop size and herein started nitrogen fixing of the soils; initially by nitrogen rich plants such as clover, and then the development of chemical fertilisers. Although this development was welcomed, it marks a key change in agriculture from sustainable and organic practices to energy intensive inputs which are dependent on the exploitation of fossil fuels.

These methods of intensive farming harm the soil by depleting the mineral stores, reducing natural organic matter, promoting soil erosion, and disrupting the natural microbial diversity of the soil. Each of which culminates in crops with a declining nutrient profile year on year. Climate change is considered to bring about further disadvantages for farming in the form of water shortages, an increase in weather variations and a rise in temperatures. In addition, higher carbon dioxide levels are considered to reduce protein, vitamin and mineral concentrations but increase growth rate and water efficiency within the plant.

Essential Minerals

Mineral losses

Micronutrient deficiencies afflict two billion people worldwide and although there are several contributing factors to worldwide malnutrition, the reducing nutrient profile of crops is a significant contributor. The mineral losses of vegetables in the UK between 1941 and 1991, showed some surprising results.

- In vegetables, the biggest losses were found in copper 75%, sodium 48% and calcium 46%,
- All the minerals except for potassium and phosphorous had losses that exceeded 20%.

- Fruit had fewer losses than vegetables, the worst hit were sodium 29%, iron 23% and copper 20%,
- All the minerals except for phosphorous had losses that exceeded 10%.

Consequently, these losses have further contributed to the negative effects of the Western diet. Combined with the increase in processed meals, simple carbohydrate foods and refined oils, nutrient deficient cheap plants further the potential malnourishment.

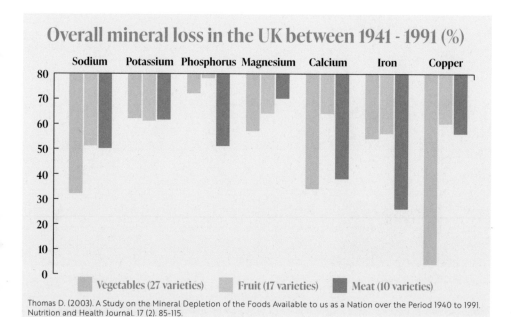

Overall mineral loss in the UK between 1941 - 1991 (%)

Vegetables (27 varieties)　Fruit (17 varieties)　Meat (10 varieties)

Thomas D. (2003). A Study on the Mineral Depletion of the Foods Available to us as a Nation over the Period 1940 to 1991. Nutrition and Health Journal. 17 (2). 85-115.

Mineral loss in meat, fruit and vegetables

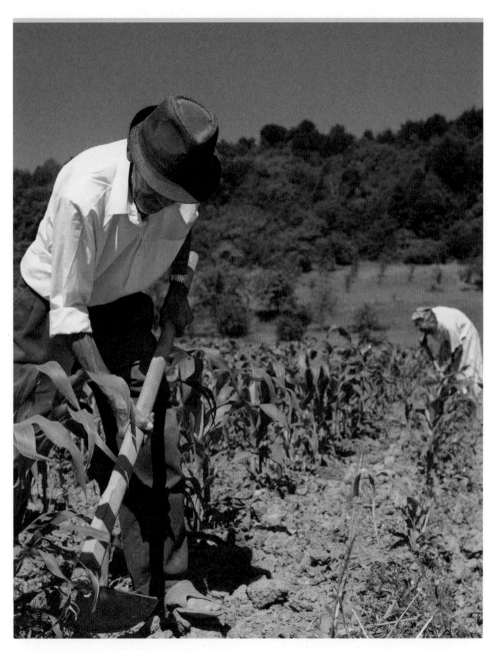

Traditional farming, such as organic, supports soil mineral stores, maintains natural organic matter, reduces soil erosion, and promotes the natural microbial diversity of the soil.

As reviewed in the previous chapter, an inadequate intake of micronutrients can be further exacerbated by health conditions, illnesses and genetics. The final piece of the puzzle lies in the activity of the human gastrointestinal tract, for instance, the tract may promote excess nutrient losses which are common in conditions such as irritable bowel disease (diarrhoea that causes an increase in intestinal motility). However, it's not just the speed of the gastrointestinal tract it is also the function. Malabsorption can occur in small intestine health conditions, such as from the result of surgery to remove a section of the bowel, gastrointestinal health conditions, and ulceration, each of which reduce the capacity for nutrients to pass through the intestinal tissues into the blood stream for passage to the liver for utilisation.

Liver damage, for example can alter how nutrients are transformed into their active versions and so potentially it reduces the availability of nutrients to assist body functions.

66 Magnesium has been shown to help patients recover from depression 99

Furthermore, genetic errors also impact how the body utilises nutrients. Genes can be thought of as our operating system, the genes 'program' the corresponding signalling agents, enzymes and transmitters, however it is known that certain genetic errors reduce the functionality of the 'operating system'. Therefore, maintaining a healthy gut with the right balance of bacteria is an important factor in optimal nutrition, something we will review in more detail in the next section.

The link between minerals and mental health

Mental health conditions are considered a biochemical imbalance in the brain but with emotional origins, nutrition can often be dismissed. This is contrary to the truth as nutrition can play an important role in the management of mental health conditions, and it can improve symptom severity and duration.

- Referred to as the spark of life, Magnesium plays a large role in the pathology of mental health conditions, in fact, a 7-day research trial saw patients fully recover from depression in response to 150-300mg magnesium taurate.

- Both zinc and iron play important roles in mental health. Several research articles have documented the beneficial effects of zinc that contribute to a reduction in depressive episodes.

- Iron deficiency is associated with a disturbance in infant cognitive function and fatigue, and in depression across all age groups.
- Iron and zinc are necessary for the normal function and energy provision to the brain.
- Iron and zinc also support regulation of the immune function. The interaction with the immune system is an important point as excessive brain inflammation is associated with an increased occurrence of mental health conditions.

These minerals are affected not only by soil depletion but also by the method whereby grains are polished to remove the husk and outer layers. These parts of the grain are the most nutrient dense and in addition to magnesium, zinc and iron they also provide some of the B vitamins, which too are nutrients involved in the regulation of mood, stress and brain function.

Nutrition and medication, what you need to know

The development of medical care has saved millions of lives since its inception, and medication plays an important role in managing chronic conditions. However, it is important to regularly review your prescription with your GP to ensure it is appropriate for your symptoms. Furthermore, as discussed certain medications will require a greater volume of specific nutrients to transform, utilise and detoxify. It is imperative that you work with your GP and discuss dietary change or the introduction of food supplements to your daily regimen.

Public Health England reported that in 2017 to 2018, 11.5 million adults in England (26% of the population), received one or more medicine prescriptions.

- 17% of the adult population were prescribed antidepressants
- 13% opioid pain relief
- 3% gapapentinoids, generally used for pain, anxiety and epilepsy
- 3% benzodiazepines, used to treat anxiety, insomnia and seizures
- 2% z-drugs, used for short term insomnia treatment

Nutrition can affect the body's response to drugs and vice versa. Some nutrients can enhance, delay or decrease the effectiveness of a medication. For example, cranberry, garlic, and turmeric should not be used alongside blood thinning medications as they work in a similar fashion. Similarly, chromium should not be used alongside blood glucose clearance medication. This type of contraindication is classed as additive, because the nutrients have a similar effect to the medication.

Conversely, some medications require a greater volume of specific nutrients because they can become depleted. Common nutrient depletions by medication include magnesium by proton pump inhibiting medication, B vitamins and zinc by antidepressant medication and Co-enzyme Q10 by statins.

Medications	Linked deficiencies
Antibiotics	• Sodium • Potassium • Vitamin C • Zinc
Oral Contraceptives	• Folic acid • Vitamins B2, B6, B12, C and E • Magnesium • Selenium • Zinc
Diabetes	• Vitamin B12 • Folate
Digestive Medication	• Iron • Calcium • Magnesium • Vitamins C and B12
Heart	• Potassium
Statins	• Co-enzyme Q10
Steroids	• Calcium • Vitamin D

Many common medications are linked to nutrient deficiencies.

To avoid contraindications, ensure you discuss any potential supplementation for these deficiencies with your GP.

Another factor to consider is fibre, whether it is fibre rich foods or supplements. Fibre can bind medications and nutrients and reduce the absorption of these compounds. This can mean that the medication does not work at the predicted dose and nutrient insufficiency may be exacerbated.

There are some cases when a health condition may be managed by optimising nutrition. This is in no way encouragement to stop medication, but purely an avenue to explore with your healthcare professional.

A prime example lies in the interesting findings that were published by Dr Dave Unwin, a GP who introduced a low carbohydrate diet for patients at his surgery that had Type II Diabetes.

Over a 6-year period where patients spent on average 23 months following a low carb diet, he reported a significant reduction in body weight and glycated haemoglobin (HbA1c) in diabetic and prediabetic patients.

Furthermore, 46% of the patients managed to reverse the diabetes without any prescription drugs. In his surgery there has been a gradual reduction in glucose regulating medication for Type II Diabetes which has resulted in a prescribing budget far lower than the average for the area.

> " Dr Dave Unwin reported that 46% of his Type II Diabetes patients reversed their condition in response to a low carbohydrate diet "

This is certainly food for thought and presents the potential for diet to help both individuals and the system as a whole. Hold that thought, as in the next section we will discuss nutrient dense foods and food supplements.

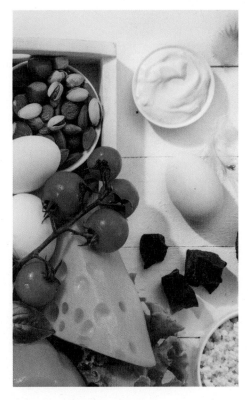

Optimising Nutrition

To consider our eating habits it can be useful to look at shopping behaviours. Data published by the Public Health Nutrition Group reported that 50.7% of the weekly supermarket shop is spent on processed foods in the UK. This means that the remaining proportion is split between household goods, non-consumables and fresh or frozen foods.

Ideally processed foods would account for no more than 20%, which would show that the population were following the 80/20 rule, whereby 80% of food intake is from wholefoods.

> " More than half the value of the weekly shop is spent on processed foods in the UK "

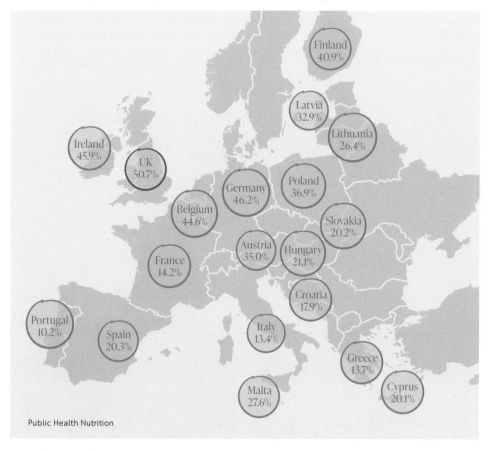

Finland 40.9%

Latvia 32.9%

Lithuania 26.4%

Ireland 45.9%

UK 50.7%

Germany 46.2%

Poland 36.9%

Belgium 44.6%

Slovakia 20.2%

Austria 35.0%

Hungary 21.1%

France 14.2%

Croatia 17.9%

Portugal 10.2%

Spain 20.3%

Italy 13.4%

Greece 13.7%

Cyprus 20.1%

Malta 27.6%

Public Health Nutrition

The UK spends more on processed food than most EU countries

It can be difficult to know where to start when making healthy food choices, not least with all the tempting offers at the supermarket and the need to find convenient and quick foods. We've seen in a previous chapter that dividing a plate into sections can give a useful guide.

- Fill half of the plate with vegetables and salad items, for example, broccoli, cauliflower, sugar snap peas, spinach, watercress, leaves, herbs, fennel, celery, peppers, cucumber, courgette, etc.

- Fill one quarter with root vegetables, such as carrots, turnips, beetroot, parsnips, etc., and potatoes, wholegrains, fruit or legumes.

- Fill the final quarter with protein (fish, meat, eggs, dairy, poultry, legumes, tofu or game).

- Add to this basic formula one tablespoon of seeds, nuts or olive oil for additional healthy fats.

- Complement with supplements tailored to your needs

- This guide can be used for every meal that is consumed from breakfast through to evening.

Another useful tool to help encourage variety is a fruit and vegetable chart categorised by colour. Each column in the chart below represents foods that are of the same colour.

For example, red = tomatoes, red apples, red peppers, berries. The idea is that on each day you tick off the food colours that have been consumed, with the goal to eat at least one item, ideally two from each colour.

Colour	Monday to Sunday
Red	Tomatoes, peppers, red onions, red lettuce, red apples, strawberries, raspberries, fresh cranberries, red grapes
Yellow / White	Peppers, bananas, lemons, pears, melon, onions, garlic, cauliflower, white cabbage, sweetcorn
Green	Salad leaves, celery, peppers, broccoli, herbs, lettuce, beans, peas, apples, grapes
Orange	Oranges, peaches, apricots, mango, squash, pumpkin, carrots, sweet potato
Purple / Blue	Blueberries, blackberries, blackcurrants, beetroot purple carrots, aubergine, grapes, cabbage

Abundant key minerals

Minerals are vital to support a healthy lifestyle. A good dietary supply of minerals can support heart function especially blood pressure, and are necessary to produce hormones and neurotransmitters (signalling agents) among other benefits such as energy production, muscle relaxation, and immunity.

As we have seen in a previous chapter, the mineral content of food is decreasing. However several foods are known for their abundance in nutrients, especially minerals, these include kelp, spirulina and chlorella. Kelp is a type of seaweed that 'grabs' nutrients from its surroundings. Subsequently it is estimated that kelp may provide over 70 different trace elements, these include, boron, calcium, copper, iron and potassium, besides magnesium, manganese and zinc.

Soil Association certified organic kelp is raised on the West coast of Ireland and Iceland. These locations have pristine and pollutant free waters due to oceanic currents and the farmers use sustainable, sea life friendly harvesting practices.

Spirulina and Chlorella are algae, they too are best when Soil Association certified organic. These freshwater algae are rich in minerals, with similar characteristics to kelp they absorb minerals from the water. Therefore, they provide a great source of iron, magnesium, potassium, copper and manganese. Plus, as a powder they make a nutritious addition to smoothies.

Other good sources of minerals include leafy green vegetables, nuts, seeds and cruciferous vegetables (Brassicas such as cauliflower, cabbage, kale, broccoli, Brussels sprouts, mustard plant and similar green leaf vegetables) as well as shellfish, cacao, and beans.

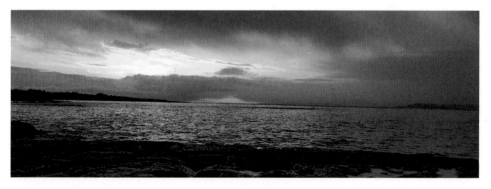

Organic kelp is raised on the West coast of Ireland

On the whole, plants are rich in minerals:

- Cruciferous vegetables, for example are rich in sulphur, magnesium, potassium and manganese, a great reason to eat broccoli, cauliflower and kale.
- Highly pigmented berries are sources of potassium, magnesium and manganese.
- Nuts and seeds are especially rich in copper, magnesium, manganese, selenium and zinc. For example, Brazil nuts are a rich source of selenium, in fact just 4-5 provide more than the daily minimum intake.
- Similarly, legumes (beans and pulses) are rich in calcium, magnesium, and iron besides potassium and copper, however certain classifications of legumes, such as beans contain phytic acid and so, it is important to soak or sprout them before cooking.
- Foods such as shellfish and eggs are rich in minerals especially zinc, selenium and iron. Highly important for energy, immunity and brain function.

When selecting mineral rich foods, look for brightly coloured plants, fruit, and plump nuts and seeds, free from dark marks, damage or dryness.

Is food enough?

For a person in good health, eating a diet that is rich in minerals that incorporates at least three or more servings of the foods listed above at each meal may be enough to provide the necessary nutrition to support health. However, this takes planning, and difficulties may arise due to family commitments, working hours and travel.

For individuals managing a health condition, mineral requirements are going to be greater than usual. This will be reflected in the required nourishment and so the quality and volume of minerals will need to be greater. Quality of life and physical capability can become a factor in ill health and the ability to prepare and cook meals can become restricted. Additionally these people may rely on meal services for food which are notoriously low quality.

In addition to time and planning, taste is a factor, people have likes and dislikes. Besides allergies and intolerances, the enjoyment or dislike of a food will play a role and can be a barrier to a mineral rich diet. Food aversion can develop based on a childhood experience and often people never revisit a disliked food, therefore reducing food choice.

Similarly, a food intolerance or food allergy to the most common allergens, namely, gluten, lactose, soy, nut, fish and shellfish can reduce the selection of mineral rich food options.

A person's surroundings can influence eating behaviour, for example, vegetables can be difficult to access for campus-based university students, additionally, travel, and location affect access to healthful food. But also, visual cues and marketing materials have a role in food selection, for example, easy access to fast food and advertising will influence food choice.

Subsequently, food is enough for healthy people taking the time to plan and follow a nutrient dense eating pattern but not necessarily for those with limited time to prepare and cook using wholefoods, as well as those suffering illnesses, those still growing and developing, pregnant or regular exercisers. Additionally the significant reduction in nutrient density of foods plays a factor in how much nutrition people can get from their diet.

	Males	Females
Vitamin A	700ug	600ug
Thiamin	1.0mg	0.8mg
Riboflavin	1.3mg	1.1mg
Niacin equivalent	16.5mg	13.2mg
Vitamin B6	1.4mg	1.2mg
Vitamin B12	1.5ug	1.5ug
Folate	200ug	200ug
Vitamin C	40mg	40mg
Vitamin D	10ug	10ug
Iron	8.7mg	14.8mg (19-50yrs) 8.7mg (50-64yrs)
Calcium	700mg	700mg
Magnesium	300mg	270mg
Potassium	3500mg	3500mg
Zinc	9.5mg	7.0mg
Copper	1.2mg	1.2mg
Iodine	140ug	140ug
Selenium	75ug	60ug
Phosphorus	550mg	550mg
Chloride	2500mg	2500mg
Sodium	2.4g	2.4g

UK Recommended intake levels of key micro nutrients for an average adult (19-64 years), but these levels only prevent deficiency, more may be required for optimum nutrition.

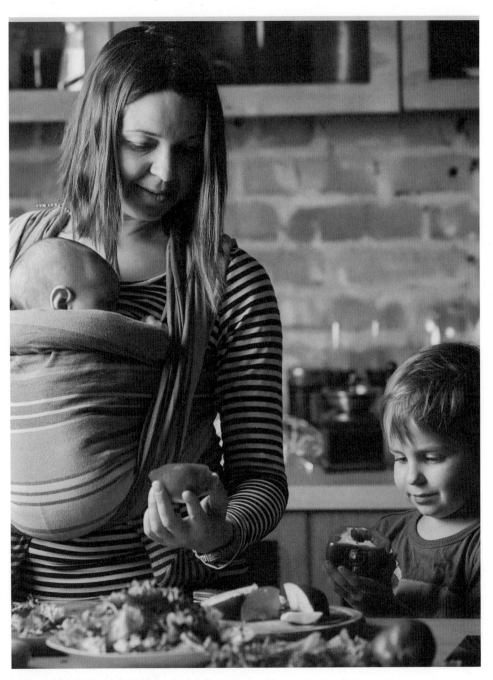

Time restrictions mean diet often suffers.

Should we consider supplementation and why?

The Scientific Advisory Committee on Nutrition advises the UK government on diet and health. They have formulated Dietary Reference Values which are a series of estimates on the energy and nutritional requirements of different groups of healthy people in the UK. Within this classification lie the Reference Nutrient Intakes (RNI) which is the amount of a nutrient that is enough to ensure the needs of 97.5% of a group are met, assuming there are no deficiencies to start with. Certain nutrients do not attract an RNI, consequently a 'Safe Intake' is set, this is the case for omega-3 essential fatty acids.

Consuming a rainbow selection of plants daily is a great start and assists a balanced wholefoods diet to provide essential nutrients such as fibre, plant specific nutrients known as phytonutrients, as well as vitamins, minerals and trace elements. However it may not contain enough nutrients and additionally, may not support the dietary needs associated with daily stress, energy requirements and times of infection or illness.

Supplementing a healthy diet with a multivitamin may therefore be beneficial. A multivitamin is a formulation of all the vitamins, minerals and trace elements that are considered essential for health. Several research papers have reported beneficial effects of a multivitamin on different health conditions such as cognition in those with mild cognitive impairment, blood pressure in hypertension patients and cardiovascular outcomes in cardiovascular disease patients.

It is important to note that a food first approach cannot be stressed enough because health maintenance cannot be achieved through a junk food diet and supplements. Food supplements purely provide extra nutrition to top up a diverse diet and support intake.

When to consider a multivitamin?

Evidence from research shows that multivitamins can address multiple nutrient insufficiencies, and so, they may be beneficial to certain groups within the population, in particular, those that cannot obtain all the necessary nutrition from their diet and are not able to adapt to do so.

Although eating a balanced diet that includes vegetables, salad items, fruit, legumes (beans and pulses), wholegrains, protein sources and healthy fats should provide healthy individuals with most of the nutrients needed for good health, it is clear from the National Diet and Nutrition Survey that many people living in Great Britain get less than the adequate amounts. Commonly, for example, people living in the UK will struggle to get enough vitamin D from food alone, the lack of which in our diets is evidenced by the rise of Rickets. In addition, those that follow restrictive eating patterns, for example, the vegan diet would need to supplement with vitamin B12, vitamin D and possibly iodine, iron, choline and calcium. Similarly, those following a keto eating pattern may struggle to consume sufficient vitamin C, folate and calcium, besides zinc and magnesium.

Public Health England recommends that everyone (including pregnant and breastfeeding women) should consider taking a daily supplement containing at least 10 micrograms (400IU) of vitamin D during the autumn and winter months.

Some groups of the population are at greater risk of not getting enough vitamin D and are advised to take a supplement every day of the year.

- breastfed babies should be given a daily supplement containing 8.5 to 10 micrograms of vitamin D from birth, even if the mother is taking a supplement containing vitamin D herself
- babies having 500mls (about a pint) or more of formula a day should not be given a vitamin D supplement, because infant formula is fortified with vitamin D and other nutrients
- all children aged 1 to 4 years old should be given a daily supplement containing 10 micrograms of vitamin D
- people who are not often exposed to the sun – such as invividuals who are frail or housebound, or usually wear clothes that cover most of their skin when outdoors - should take a daily supplement containing at least 10 micrograms of vitamin D

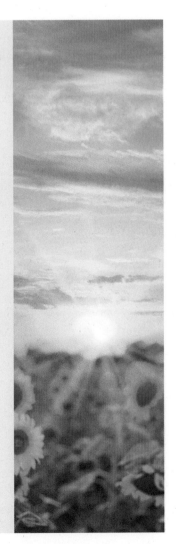

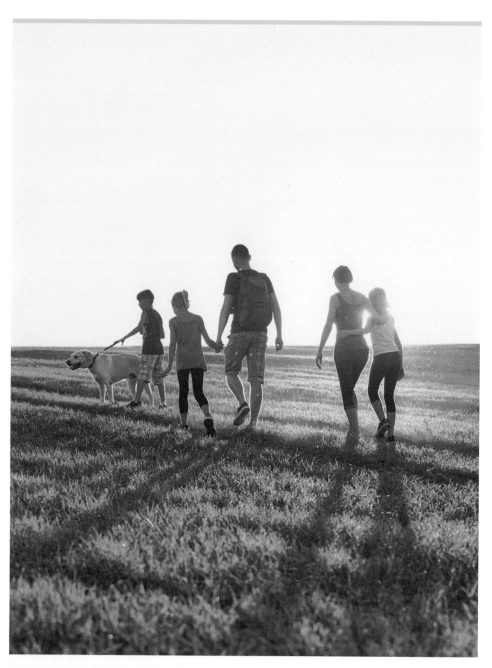

Vitamin D is obtained through sun exposure and some foods but many people in the UK are deficient

Diseases that are caused by a lack of specific dietary nutrients include scurvy (vitamin C), beri-beri (vitamin B1), pellagra (vitamin B3) and rickets (vitamin D). Other conditions to consider supplementation include those where deficiencies are caused by long term poor nutrition or malabsorption through poor digestive health.

Other groups within the population that are at risk of nutrient insufficiencies:

- **Elderly**
  The elderly can be at risk of nutrient insufficiencies due to physical difficulties such as difficulty chewing and swallowing foods, time spent indoors, alteration of taste in response to medications plus isolation and loneliness can suppress the appetite. In addition, the gastric secretions necessary for the absorption of vitamin B12 decrease with age and medications can reduce nutrients available in the body.
- **Pregnancy and lactation**
  There is a strong association between poor folate intake and the development of neural tube defects in the foetus. Subsequently, folic acid supplementation is encouraged in preparation for pregnancy. However, some pregnancies are unplanned and so Public Health England recommend that all women of childbearing age supplement with 400mcg of folic acid daily. In addition, upon pregnancy and throughout lactation additional iron, calcium, vitamin D, iodine and the omega-3 essential fatty acid docosahexaenoic acid (DHA) is needed by the body to form and support the baby. In fact, suboptimal levels of DHA have been associated with postpartum depression.

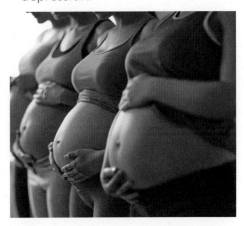

Additional iron, calcium, vitamin D, iodine and omega-3 essential fatty acids are needed during pregnancy to form and support the baby

- **Malabsorption conditions**
  A health condition that interferes with digestion may contribute to nutrient insufficiencies. For example, coeliac disease, colitis, Crohn's disease and inflammatory bowel diseases.

However, surgical interventions too influence absorption, such as gastric bypass or bowel resection. Finally, alcohol has been found to prevent several B vitamins and vitamin C absorption.

- **Taking certain medication**
Certain diuretic medications which increase urination are known to deplete the body of magnesium, zinc, potassium and calcium. Plus, proton pump inhibitors that alkalise the digestive tract to prevent acid reflux can deplete the body of magnesium and prevent the absorption of B vitamins, especially folate, B6 and B12.

In addition, 2019 Kantar research suggests as many as 38% of people are trying to lose weight most of the time. To gain an understanding of the nutrient intake of common weight loss diets, a study investigated the caloric and micronutrient content of typical meals prescribed for each the 'Atkins for Life' diet, South Beach diet, and the DASH diet. The results showed that these popular diet plans failed to provide the minimum recommended dietary intake for all the 27 micronutrients. In fact, a whopping 27,575 calories daily would need to be consumed to achieve micronutrient (vitamins and minerals) recommended intakes, a figure that would increase body mass drastically if consumed long term.

Furthermore, biotin, vitamin D, E, chromium, iodine and molybdenum were identified as consistently low or non-existent across the diet plans. These results show that most common diet plans may be vastly deficient in micronutrients, the risk is that organs and body systems are not supported nutritionally and good health may be compromised.

Optimising performance

When exploring sporting performance, it is considered that most physically active people consume a quantity of vitamins and minerals consistent to the recommendations for people generally. However, should their intake be less than the recommendations, research shows that performance can deteriorate. Reports show that folate and vitamin B12 insufficiency result in anaemia and reduced capacity for endurance performance. Fundamentally all mineral insufficiencies reduce performance, especially iron deficiency which reduce muscle capabilities and work capacity. Magnesium insufficiency may increase oxygen requirements during exercise and subsequently reduce endurance performance. Nutrient insufficiencies may be identified by blood tests to allow personalised treatment.

How to find a good multi

With so many different food supplements on offer it can be difficult to find an appropriate multivitamin to meet your needs.

Firstly, look for a reputable company, they will provide contact details so that you can ask questions and advice. Dig a bit deeper and ask if they are a member of the Health Food Manufacturers Association (HFMA) which ensures they comply with all regulations including Good Manufacturing Practice Code. Find out about animal testing, the ownership of the company and the use of environmentally negative ingredients like palm oil.

A reputable company will base their formulations on human research evidence, namely the findings of human clinical trials. Furthermore, a qualified nutrition professional will have formulated the supplements including the nutrients and quantities provided.

- **Avoid excipients**
  Excipients are non-nutritive substances, i.e. they have no benefit to the person taking them but are used to aid manufacture.
  - Magnesium stearate is a white, water grabbing compound that despite its name does not provide dietary magnesium. It is used as a flow agent. It grabs water from the environment so that the nutrients flow through the machines easily, whereas any form of humidity or damp would slow the flow and cause blockages.
  - Titanium dioxide is a common compound that gives tablets and capsules a uniform white colour. It is a mined compound and used in white paint. It is found in medication as well as many foodstuffs (for example, cheese, coffee creamer, icing) and should be avoided. The European Food Standards Authority recently made a recommendation for the substance to be banned in food.
  - Carrageenan is another common excipient. This is a gelling agent which comes from a type of red seaweed called Irish Moss. It sounds nice enough but when isolated from the plant matrix, it is considered highly inflammatory. Surprisingly carrageenan is not just in food supplements, it is used in milk alternatives, dairy, cottage cheese, yogurt and cream.

Food supplements made without excipients incorporate slow manufacturing practices whereby the formula is run through the machines in small quantities so that blockages do not occur, and the machine does not overheat and damage the nutrients. This process is the difference between nutrients blended with flow and bulking agents and food supplements that are 100% nutrition.

Gelatin, Sorbitol Syrup, Palm Oil, Beeswax.

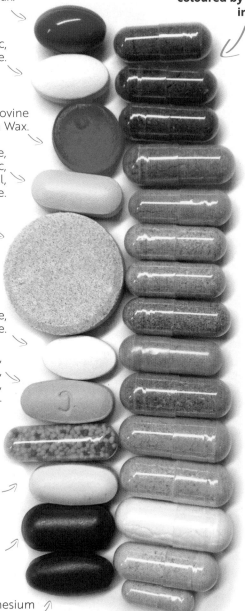

Capsules which are naturally coloured by the active ingredients

Magnesium Stearate, Talc, Titanium Dioxide, Sucrose.

Maltitol, Sucralose, Bovine Gelatine, Carmine, Carnuba Wax.

Dicalcium Phosphate, Titanium Dioxide, Purified Talc, Sugar, Sucrose, Mannitol, Magnesium Stearate.

Sorbitol, Anti Foaming Agent (Polysorbate 60), Aspartame, Acesulphate K, Mannitol.

Magnesium Stearate, Titanium Dioxide.

Gelatin, Glucose Syrup, Sucrose, Insoluble Polyvinylpyrrolidon, Magnesium Stearate, Polysorbate.

Gelatin, Shellac, Titanium Dioxide, Talc.

Di Calcium Phosphate, Magnesium Stearate, Glucose, Sucrose, Talc, Brilliant Blue, Fractionated Vegetable Oil, Glucose Syrup.

Dibasic Calcium Phosphate, Glyceril Tristearate, Magnesium Stearate, Cross-linked Cellulose Gum, Titanium Dioxide, Sucrose.

Glucose Syrup, Magnesium Stearate, Silicon Dioxide, Sucrose.

Check the label of supplements carefully for unnecessary ingredients.

One of the benefits of purchasing UK manufactured food supplements is that they must conform to strict standards in terms of contaminants, heavy metals and microbiology. But also processes such as genetic modification and irradiation must be clearly labelled.

Taking your daily multivitamin

- Choosing capsules, powders and liquids means you are likely to avoid the most common excipients. Almost all tablets contain glues and binders
- Take supplements with food to aid absorption
- Use water to swallow capsules
- Some capsules can be opened and mixed with food/smoothies but check the label first
- Do not add supplements to hot food as it is likely to denature the vitamins
- Take fat soluble vitamins (e.g. vitamin D and E) with healthy fat foods such as avocado or oily fish
- Beware of anti-nutrients – some foods can limit the absorption of nutrients.
- Tannins found in tea are known to block the absorption of iron

How to measure a vitamin or mineral

Gram
1 g=1000mg

A gram is a metric measurement of weight. An old imperial measure of weight is the ounce.
1 ounce = 28.4 grams

⇩

Milli gram
1 mg=1000mcg

One milligram is one thousandth of a gram and one thousand micrograms. A milligram is generally abbreviated as mg.

⇩

Micro gram

One microgram is one millionth of a gram and one thousandth of a milligram. It is usually abbreviated as mcg or µg (they're the same).

But what about IU?

The IU is an International Unit, usually used to measure fat soluble vitamins including vitamin A, D and E. The conversion of IU to mg varies depending on the nutrient.

Vitamin A
One milligram of beta carotene = 1667IU of vitamin A activity.
15mg of beta carotene = 25,000IU of vitamin A activity.

Vitamin E
One milligram of vitamin E = approx 1.21 to 1.49IU (depending on the carrier).
400IU of d-alpha tocopherol = 268mg.

Vitamin D
One microgram of vitamin D = 40IU.
400IU of vitamin D = 10ug.

Probiotics

Get that good gut feeling

Getting all the right nutrients for your life stage and level of health is hugely important but it isn't the only factor. The importance of gut health is sometimes underestimated, yet we need good digestive health to liberate nutrients from food and their subsequent absorption to fulfil multiple roles in the body.

The digestive system is both incredibly simple, but also phenomenally complex. The body needs proteins, fats, carbohydrates, vitamins and minerals plus water. In basic terms, foods and drinks are consumed, chewed and broken down by the digestive system into their component nutrients of proteins into amino acids, fats into fatty acids and glycerol, and carbohydrates into short saccharide chains.

In this section, we explore how digestion works, what can go wrong and the vital role of good gut bacteria in digestive health.

Digestive troubles

- Up to 1 in 4 people in the UK suffer from irritable bowel syndrome
- Another 1 in 4 suffer from chronic constipation - with many using stimulant laxatives
- The prevalence of dyspepsia in the general population has been estimated to be 20-40%

The digestive process

Digestion starts with thoughts of food. You will be familiar with how food aromas give you a sensation of hunger, prompt the production of salvia and trigger gastric secretions which can lead to a rumbling tummy. The production of acidic fluids in the stomach activates digestive enzymes.

Foods travel from the mouth down the oesophagus to the stomach, where the foods mix with digestive acids, to the small intestine, interacting with the pancreas and liver, and into the large intestine and beyond where the waste is finally expelled.

Food is transported via a process called peristalsis, whereby layers of muscle throughout the gastro-intestinal tract enable the walls to move and squeeze the food forward through the system.

Once in the small intestine, additional enzymes provided by the pancreas and liver, enable the walls to absorb water and take the digested nutrients into the bloodstream.

The large intestine absorbs more water and transports the waste further down the digestive system into the rectum ready for a bowel movement. The entire process is governed by our hormones and central nervous system.

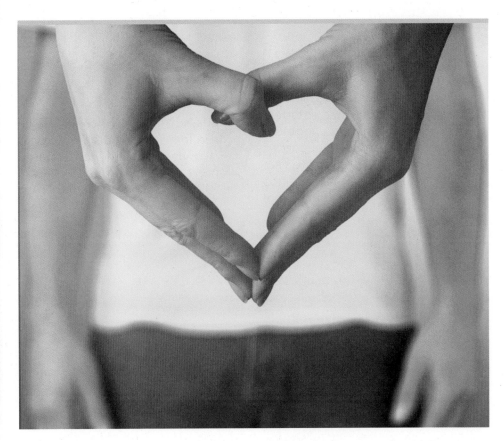

Gut-brain axis

It may sound bizarre that the digestive tract and the brain are in constant communication, but it is true. The phrases 'gut feeling' or 'gut instinct' both stem from this relationship. The communication is between the central nervous system that transmits messages from the brain via the spinal cord, and the enteric nervous system, which is the primary nervous system of the digestive tract. This links emotional and cognitive parts of the brain to digestive function.

Messages are sent in both directions via hormones, brain cells, immune cells, and the microbiome. This may explain the link between pathogenic bacterial dominance of the microbiome and mental health conditions. For instance, it is well known that irritable bowel syndrome (IBS) is considered demonstrative of this relationship because it can involve digestive disruption, stress, anxiety, and mental health symptoms.

Just Can't Stomach This. When the Gut Goes Wrong.

The digestive tract is the body's primary interface between the outside world and our organs, tissues and the bloodstream. Here food, pathogens (bacteria, virus, fungi), chemicals, metals and hormones are either absorbed, repelled, or cling to tissue.

With such a large exposure risk, the digestive tract has an abundance of immune cells to defend the body and prevent these substances from crossing into the bloodstream.

How substances are dealt with is based on immune strength and classification. For example, if the perception is that a substance is a 'friend' it will be allowed to be absorbed and repelled if 'foe'. However, if immunity is weak and undernourished, this increases the risk of an infection or toxicity as the immune function does not have the necessary resources to work optimally.

In the detection of a food allergen, toxin or bacteria, the cells within the tissues may move apart as part of an alarm response and if they do not reunite, their integrity is compromised, often referred to as a 'leaky gut'.

The importance of gut health is sometimes underestimated, as we need good digestive health to liberate nutrients from food and their subsequent absorption to fulfil multiple roles in the body. Without this function we would become fatally malnourished.

Malfunctions of digestive health

Malnourishment, genetics, infection, stress and lifestyle choices can impact on the health of the digestive system. Primary conditions include:

- Acid reflux
- Coeliac disease
- Colitis
- Constipation
- Crohn's disease
- Diarrhoea
- Diverticular disease
- Dyspepsia (indigestion)
- Haemorrhoids
- Irritable bowel
- Leaky gut

Correct diagnosis by a qualified practitioner is essential, and specific diet and supplement advice for each condition can be found in your local independent health food store.

What are probiotics?

It may be unfamiliar to think of bacteria as beneficial because we know all too well that bacteria can cause infections and illness. Yet some bacterial strains are highly beneficial for health and can contribute to health improvements. These are beneficial-gut bacteria and known as probiotics. Certain yeasts can also function as probiotics.

Beneficial bacteria produce short chain fatty acids from the fermentation of prebiotic fibres, these fatty acids instruct beneficial functions in the body such as immune support, glucose management, reduction of gut pH and support of the mucosal barrier function, these are the cells that line the small intestine. They even help to manufacture certain B vitamins and vitamin K2.

When a baby is born, the digestive tract is sterile, bacteria are transferred from the mother during the journey down the birth canal, while breastfeeding and during skin-to-skin contact. The bacteria colonise the gut and the microbiome is formed. So important is this proliferation of bacteria, it is considered by many to be an organ of the body.

The microbiome evolves as the child develops into adulthood but can be compromised by limited and poor food choices, antibiotic use and other lifestyle choices such as excessive sanitation, alcohol and smoking.

Where have all the good bugs gone?

Digestive health has been impacted by the industrial revolution and the increase in urbanised living.

As we've seen in previous sections, the change in diet and lifestyle has resulted in the increase of non-communicable disease (e.g diabetes) and when it comes to digestive health the prevalence of gastrointestinal conditions is known to be increasing. Factors that have reduced good gut bacteria and increased bad bacteria include making limited food choices, antibiotic overuse (both supplied in foods, and as medications) and the lack of dietary fibre.

What's in a name?

These are all different terms for describing the good gut bacteria found mostly in the large intestine (colon):

- Probiotics
- Gut flora
- Microbiota
- Microbiome

The good vs the bad

There are many trillions of bacteria in the human body, and thousands of different bacterial strains. Often we think of bacteria as bad but this isn't always the case. You'll be familiar with names such as *streptococcus, escherichia coli* and *salmonella*, which when out of control are associated with pneumonia, meningitis, food poisoning and more. We need small amounts of these bacteria for normal functioning of the microbiome. It is when their colonies become large that they are a problem and exert negative effects on health.

The best-researched and most commonly available probiotic supplements include *Lactobacillus* and *Bifidobacterium* Strains.

Probiotic supplement strains

- *Lactobacillus acidophilus*
- *Lactobacillus rhamnosus GG*
- *Bifidobacterium breve*
- *Bifidobacterium infantis*
- *Bifidobacterium longum*
- *Bifidobacterium lactis*
- *Bifidobacterium bifidum*
- *Bifidobacterium animalis*
- *Saccharomyces boulardii* (a yeast with probiotic properties)

Individually, and in varied combinations, there is a wealth of research to indicate their beneficial effects in a wide range of health conditions.

The term 'probiotic' arose from the Latin work 'pro' meaning 'for' and the Greek word 'bios', for life.

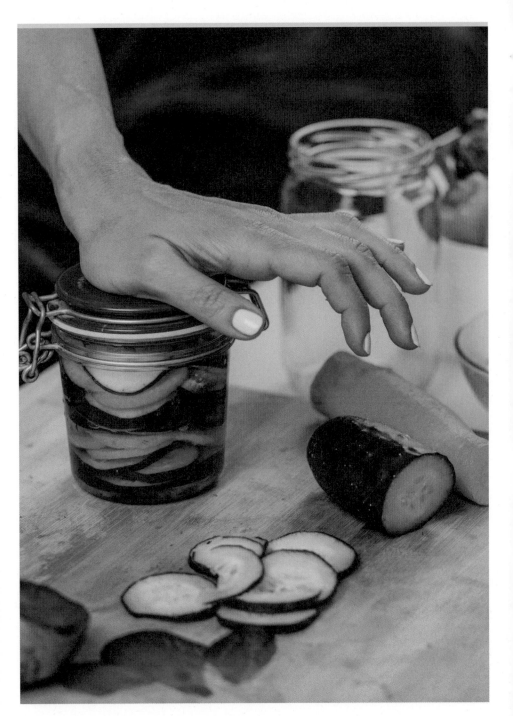

What are prebiotics and synbiotics?

It can be common to see probiotics blended with prebiotic fibres, these are known as synbiotics.

Prebiotics are foods (typically high-fibre foods) that act as food for the microflora. The microbiome feeds upon the resistant fibres. You'll find all these and more in your local specialist health food store, with advice of how to incorporate them into your lifestyle.

Prebiotic vs probiotic

Probiotics are the live beneficial bacteria

Prebiotics are a food source for the beneficial bacteria

Good gut food choices
Foods rich in probiotics
• Fermented foods
• Live yoghurt
• Kefir
• Sauerkraut
• Tempeh
• Kimchi
• Miso
• Kombucha
• Natto
Foods rich in prebiotics
• Fibrous fruits e.g. unripe bananas, apples
• Vegetables e.g. chicory, jerusalem artichoke
• Whole grains

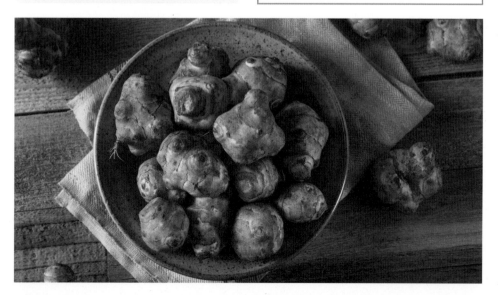

The benefits of bacteria

Research into beneficial bacteria is highly dynamic and new findings are published regularly. There are several instances to evidence the beneficial activity of 'friendly' bacteria.

- **Antibiotic-related diarrhoea**
  This can be a common side effect of antibiotic therapy as the medication alters the microbiome. Evidence shows relief of antibiotic-associated diarrhoea in response to supplementation with the beneficial yeast *Saccharomyces boulardii* or *Lactobacillus rhamnosus GG*.

- **Infectious diarrhoea**
  Research has shown improvements in response to *Saccharomyces boulardii* and *Lactobacillus rhamnosus GG*.

- **Allergies / Eczema / Asthma**
  Compelling evidence shows that allergies, eczema and asthma improve in response to *Lactobacillus rhamnosus GG* and *Bifidobacterium lactis*.

- **Natural antibiotic action**
  Several bacterial strains appear to produce antibiotic-like substances, for example *Lactobacillus acidophillus* is known to produce such a substance called acidophillin, subsequently these compounds are highly beneficial in supporting the immune system.

- **Urinary tract**
  Combining cranberry extract with *Lactobacillus acidophilus*. Research has shown that the *lactobacilli* species dominate the urogenital flora of healthy premenopausal women, therefore it is suggested that the restoration of the urogenital flora with *lactobacilli*, when in a state of infection, may protect against urinary tract infections.

- **Brain/mental health**
  Early research is promising in the creation of a category called 'psychobiotics' which may have application in low mood and depression.

- **Constipation**
  Although several factors may play a role in the onset of constipation such as a sedentary lifestyle, fluid intake and fibre intake, interesting evidence has been reported for the use of beneficial bacteria, these include *Bifidobacterium bifidum*, *Bifidobacterium longum*, *Lactobacillus rhamnosus GG* and *Lactobacillus acidophilus*.

- **IBS**
  Various strains of bacteria have proved helpful in this syndrome including *Bifidobacterium bifidum*, *Lactobacillus rhamnosus*, *Lactobacillus animalis*, *Lactobacillus acidophilus*, *Bifidobacterium infantis* and *Saccharomyces bouldardii*.

Side effects / contraindications

Probiotics and prebiotics are generally well tolerated. But there are circumstances when they are not recommended. Those with conditions that involve a weakened immune system such as HIV, AIDS or those undergoing cancer treatment, should take advice from a healthcare professional.

If taking a probiotic for the first time be aware of the Herxheimer effect. Commonly called 'die off', it is when new bacteria are introduced to the digestive tract and colonies of infectious bacteria naturally die off. The infectious bacteria are quite toxic and so their death may cause a little abdominal discomfort, bloating or gas, possible looseness, or diarrhoea. It is recommended that if you are new to probiotics or if you have gastrointestinal upset, to start the beneficial bacteria when you are at home. Generally, the Herxheimer effect ends after to 5-7 days while the colonies of bacteria adapt to the supplementation.

Digestive dangers

Substances to avoid to reduce the load on the digestive tract:
- Additives
- Emulsifiers
- Synthetic flavours
- Synthetic colours

7 steps for choosing the most effective probiotics

1. Choose a pure supplement with no excipients, as unnecessary additives may potentially inflame or burden the gut.
2. Look for the bacterial strain which should be listed on the label by a letter-number code.
3. The formula may include a prebiotic alongside the probiotics, such as FOS or plant-derived inulin.
4. Choose a capsule or powder form to ease a compromised digestion.
5. Packaged in glass for protection from light, but no need for refrigeration.
6. At least 1 billion viable microorganisms per capsule/ serving.
7. Look for an age-appropriate supplement
   - Pregnancy
   - Infants and babies
   - Children
   - 40+

Fats Are Good For You!

Over the decades, the role and benefits of fats have been controversial. The root of confusion is derived from poorly conducted research which has also been incorrectly interpreted into public health messages. For many years the conclusions were not challenged or cross checked and, in the meantime, the public were told that fats were bad for health. Luckily, some outspoken researchers challenged these beliefs which lead to a flurry of investigative research into the effects of fats in each of their forms, namely saturated, monounsaturated, polyunsaturated, and trans-fats. In this chapter, we'll discover how essential fat is for our health and how best to incorporate good fats into our daily diet.

The great fat fast

In the 1980's and 1990's we were told to avoid fats altogether. It was believed that fats made us gain weight and contributed to cardiovascular illnesses. Many people removed all natural fats from their diets and replaced with vegetable fats including margarine and those found in highly processed foods (trans-fats), thinking they were investing in their health.

Spreading truth

The truth is that fat is essential to a healthy life. We need fats for hormone production, to make cells, to quell inflammation and support energy production.

However, it is of great importance that foods with beneficial fats are selected. And herein lies the source of the confusion over fats and their effect on health.

What are fats?

Fat is a macronutrient, a term that is reflective of its large molecular size. However, a subsection of fats includes essential fatty acids. These fatty acids are termed essential as the body cannot make them, and so they must come from the diet. Fats are found in animal-derived foods (meat, dairy, eggs) and also in plant-based foods (nuts, seeds and even in some vegetables).

It's useful to know that foods provide several forms of fat: saturated, monounsaturated (MUFA), polyunsaturated (PUFA) and the most dangerous, trans-fats.

Foods generally contain several forms of fat. For example, walnuts provide MUFAs, PUFAs and saturated fats. Therefore, a food always provides several fat types and never just one type of fat in isolation.

What's in a Name?

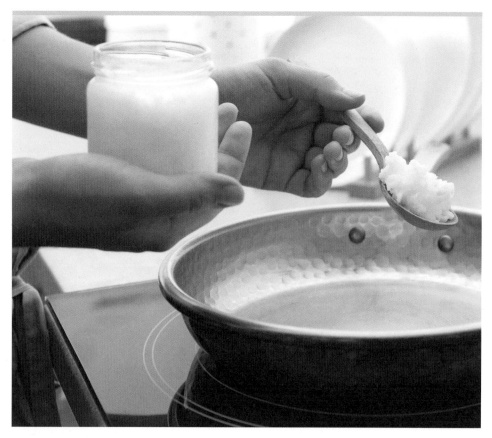

Essential fatty acids (EFAs), omega-3, 6, 7 & 9 or nutritional oils – these are all ways to describe the important fats that can be consumed as foods or added as a food supplement.

Saturated fat

Named so as each carbon molecule is 'saturated' with hydrogen molecules. A quick and easy way of identifying when a food is predominantly saturated fat is if the food is solid at room temperature. For example, cheese, animal fat, coconut oil, butter.

This type of fat is structurally strong and makes a great fat for cooking and baking. Saturated fat is transformed into cholesterol, which is then transformed into hormones. Subsequently, it is important to include a small amount of saturated fat in the diet so that testosterone and oestrogen among other hormones can be produced.

A lack thereof can lead to poor skin health, brain fog, and infertility besides changes in appetite and the inability to cope with stress.

Conversely too much saturated fat has been associated with elevated cholesterol which is a risk of oxidative damage and ultimately can contribute to cardiovascular health conditions.

It is generally considered that 20 and 30 grams of saturated fats for females and males respectively is the optimal amount.

Unsaturated fat

You have guessed it, not every carbon molecule is 'saturated' with hydrogen molecules.
Unsaturated fats fall into two categories: polyunsaturated fatty acids and monounsaturated fatty acids, referred to as PUFAs and MUFAs and both are liquid at room temperature.

MUFAs are present in avocado, nuts and olives. It is considered that MUFAs can help to modulate cholesterol type. For example, Low Density Lipoprotein Cholesterol (LDL-C) is often considered 'bad', and High-Density Lipoprotein Cholesterol (HDL-C) considered 'good'.

LDL-C is cholesterol that is being shuttled out to cells and tissue, it is at a high risk of oxidative damage, and this is when it is of detriment to health, thus labelled 'bad'. HDL-C is cholesterol that is being shuttled to the liver and ultimately will leave the body, hence referred to as good.

It is deemed that the optimal scenario is when LDL-C is low and HDL-C is higher, which is purported to occur when saturated fats are decreased and MUFAs increased, however we cannot ignore that total cholesterol too is important. PUFAs are present in sunflower seeds, sesame seeds and seafood. Similarly, reducing saturated fat intake and increasing PUFA intake is considered to reduce LDL-C. PUFAs are split into two types, omega-3 and omega-6 essential fatty acids.

Trans-fats

A hydrogenated fat or oil.
This can be any type of fat that has been heated until the bonds between the molecules break and upon cooling, they then bond again but into a different formation. The process is called hydrogenation when completed in a commercial setting, but trans fats can be produced when fragile fats are heated, which in general can occur when seed fats are used for high temperature cooking.

To avoid hydrogenated fats, you can check the label when purchasing cooking oils and avoid those that state hydrogenised fats or partially hydrogenised oil. Trans-fats are highly damaging to health, and it is considered that they can enter the cell and damage DNA, highly worrying as DNA is the programming code for every body function.

Due to this risk, Public Health England recommends that total trans-fat intake does not exceed 2% of total energy intake. To put this into perspective; if a person requires 2000 calories daily to function and maintain their current body composition (fat, muscle and bone proportions), 2% of intake is 40 calories.

Trans-fats are 9 calories per gram; therefore 40 calories equates to 4.4 grams, which is less than a teaspoon. Now that emphasises how dangerous trans-fats may potentially be!

Subsequently, processed foods produced in the UK are legally obliged to state on the nutritional panel how much trans-fat a food provides; however, this is only when the trans-fat is an ingredient. It does not include those that transform fats into trans-fat during production. Therefore, it's no surprise that the major advantage of eating a wholefood diet is that trans-fats are not present.

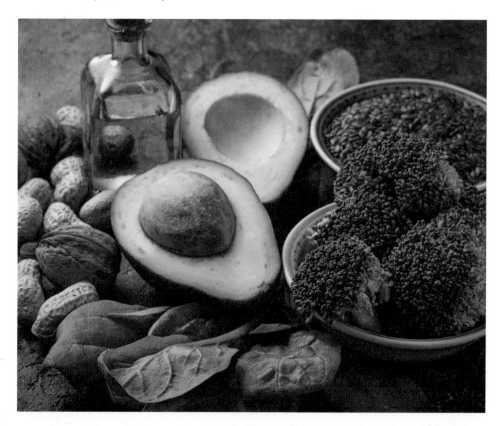

Fat by the Numbers

Understanding omega-3, 6, 7 and 9

Fatty acids are called 'omega' and then a number, for example omega-3 or omega-6 because when you look at the molecular structure at 3 or 6 carbons from the end, there appears a double bond. This is important because the human body cannot always produce a double bond and so this means the body cannot make omega-3 nor omega-6 essential fatty acids but must consume them. Hence, they are termed 'essential'.

The importance of omega-3

Omega-3 essential fatty acids are a group of fatty acids found mainly in flaxseed, perilla seed, algae, and fish. These include alpha linolenic acid (ALA) found in flaxseed and perilla seed, and the remaining eicosapentaenoic acid (EPA), docosapentaenoic acid and docosahexaenoic acid (DHA) are found in fish and algae.

Research has revealed that the most potent anti-inflammatory effects are the omega-3 forms found in fish and algae. However, upon consumption of flaxseed or perilla seed, the body can slowly transform the omega-3 fatty acids into the forms present in fish and algae to exert their anti-inflammatory and cell structure benefits. Research reports that women and infants are the most efficient at this conversion, while it is apparent that others struggle with the conversion and so it is important that they consume good amounts of fish and/or marine algae forms.

Preferred natural sources of Omegas			
Omega-3	**Omega-6**	**Omega-7**	**Omega-9**
• Flax seed	• Hemp seed	• Sea buckthorn	• Avocado
• Perilla seed	• Black seed	• Avocado	• Sunflower seeds
• Fatty fish	(*Nigella sativa*)	• Olives	• Olives
• Marine algae	• Avocado	• Macadamia nuts	• Hazelnuts
• Chia seeds	• Walnuts		• Almonds

Benefits of omega-3

- **Heart health**
  An omega-3 rich diet may support heart health by reducing blood triglycerides (fats in the blood stream), blood pressure and blood clotting. Scientists worldwide have shown interest in the effects of omega-3 essential fatty acids on human health.

- **Cholesterol**
  It is known that an omega-3 rich diet may support heart health by reducing blood triglycerides (fats in the blood stream), blood pressure and blood clotting. In addition, omega-3 essential fatty acids may promote a process called reverse cholesterol transport. This is the mechanism by which excess cholesterol from tissues are transported to the liver for excretion. This function is of primary importance for the risk reduction of atherosclerosis by the reduction of LDL-C and increase of HDL-C. A further study showed that 2g of omega-3 fish oil given twice daily for 8 weeks produced a reduction in LDL-C and increase in HDL-C.

- **Rheumatoid arthritis**
  Observational studies found a link between rheumatoid arthritis patients and low omega-3 status. Subsequently, omega-3 supplementation was shown to reduce morning stiffness, joint swelling, tenderness and pain.

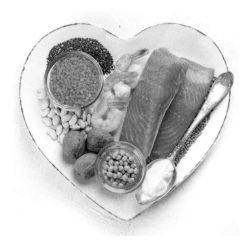

- **Skin conditions**
  Omega-3 insufficiencies have been related to eczema and other skin conditions. It was observed that omega-3 supplementation helped to alleviate dry, itchy and inflamed skin plus it reduced moisture loss.

- **Mental health**
  New theories surrounding mental health include an inflamed brain, neural circuits and central nervous system hypothesis. Studies investigating associations between omega-3 status and mental health states noted insufficiency in those with depression, bipolar disorder, dementia, cognitive impairment and behavioural and learning disorders such as dyslexia and attention deficit disorder. In addition, EPA and DHA supplementation showed benefits in treating depression and mental disorders.

- **Menopause**

  The menopausal transition can be considered highly inflammatory due to the reduction in hormone production and function of the ovaries. Subsequently several life affecting symptoms can present during this time.

  Omega-3 essential fatty acids are considered useful in the EPA and DHA forms due to their interaction with the inflammatory cascade. Subsequently a study reported a reduction in blood pressure and the inflammation marker, IL-6 in response to 900mg of omega-3 fish oils taken in addition to their regular diet for six months. Furthermore, a small study investigating depressive symptoms during the menopausal transition saw an improvement in symptom severity in response to 2g daily of omega-3 fish oils.

Further benefits of omega-3 essential fatty acids are proposed for:

- Gastrointestinal disorders
- Diabetes
- Obesity
- PMS including breast tenderness
- Blood pressure
- Asthma
- Allergies

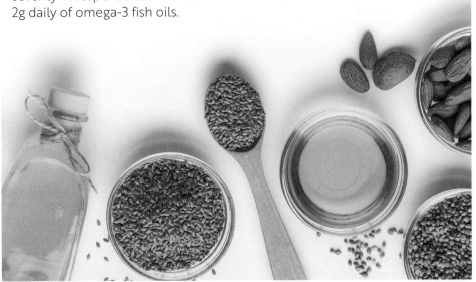

Omega-6, 7 & 9

Omega-6s are widely available in the Western diet and rarely need to be supplemented except for specific health conditions where omega-6 rich foods such as hemp or black seeds are consumed. Reducing processed foods and ensuring the prevalent source of your diet is from wholefoods, will naturally derive your omega-6 from healthier sources.

The body can manufacture omega-7 and omega-9 using MUFA's and PUFA's in the diet, however certain foods and supplements can be helpful in specific conditions such as eye health and vaginal dryness.

Omega-6:3 ratio

The omega-6:3 ratio is now considered the true marker of healthy fat consumption. Typically, the Western diet omega-6:3 ratio can be as high as 20:1, but the goal is to reduce the ratio to around 3:1. That is, no more than three parts omega-6, to one part omega-3. It is at the lower ratio that the prevention and management of chronic health conditions may be achieved.

In support, population research showed that a ratio of 4:1 was associated with a 70% decrease in death from any cause. Similarly, a ratio of approx. 3:1 suppressed inflammation in rheumatoid arthritis patients and a ratio of 5:1 improved asthma symptoms. Yet a ratio of 10:1 revealed adverse health consequences.

As mentioned previously, fat-rich wholefoods provide a range of fats, often MUFAs, PUFAs and saturated fats, therefore if the focus is on the provision of omega-3 rich foods in the diet, this will also fulfil omega-6, MUFA, PUFA and saturated fat requirements.

Reasons to up your intake of omega-3:

- For its anti-inflammatory properties from EPA and DHA
- DHA is densely found in the eye, brain and sperm cells
- To normalise elevated blood fats
- To support joint health
- To boost mood
- Essential in pregnancy and breastfeeding for infant development
- May support cognitive function such as mental skills, memory, knowledge acquisition and recall

8 steps to choose the right omega supplement for you

Fish oil is an excellent source of omega-3, EPA and DHA, but take care when selecting a fish oil supplement from supermarket shelves or online, as there is huge variation between different brands and sources. When selecting a fish oil, visit a specialist health food store and consider those that have been raised in a river environment rather than the ocean. Freshwater fish can be raised and certified Soil Association Organic if the river environment is surrounded by a minimum of 10km of land that is free from pesticides and chemical fertilisers. This naturally provides a fish oil that is not exposed to ocean contaminants and pollution.

Take care to check whether the capsule is bovine gelatin, fish gelatin or vegetable source.

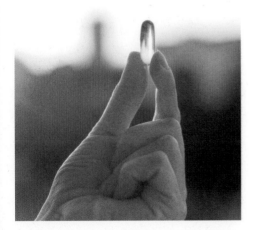

1. River-source fish oil (low pollution) provides naturally occurring omega levels found in the fish and not chemically altered to provide higher levels of omega-3.

2. Organically certified (free from artificial chemicals)

3. Excipient-free (no synthetic flavours, colours or preservatives)

4. First cold-pressed seed oils (preserves the nutrient value)

5. Liquid oils packaged under nitrogen blanket (protects against oxidization)

6. Packaged in amber glass and outer cardboard (to protect from heat and light)

7. Vegan marine algae source of EPA and/or DHA is available

8. Look for omega supplements for your life-stage or condition:
   • Pregnancy
   • Children
   • Skin health
   • Anti-ageing
   • Joint health
   • Women
   • Aged 40+

Staff in independent health food stores are knowledgeable and experienced in advising on nutritional oils to boost omega-3 intake or address specific health conditions. They will recommend the right supplement and correct daily intake for your individual needs.

Lifestyle

Eating the right foods and obtaining all the required nutrients is crucial but only part of a healthy lifestyle approach. Traditional eating methods such as the Mediterranean diet and the Blue Zones way of life acknowledge that health comes from several facets, these include, time outdoors, regular movement and the sense of community in addition to the consumption of wholefoods.

Similarly, governing health bodies recognise that dietary change is not the total solution to the health crisis, and it is proposed that a healthy lifestyle goes hand in hand with an improved dietary intake of nutrients. This proposition is supported by an observational study which investigated the contributing factors in male centenarians in Sardinia. It was observed that their longevity was highly influenced by their past lifestyle habits. Specifically, lifestyle habits that occurred in the early 20th century. In addition, physical activity and occupation activity levels also had a beneficial effect, namely, activities based on shepherding and farming the highlands of Sardinia.

Physical activity

In the UK, in recognition of a lifestyle approach to health, Public Health England recommend activity guidelines categorised by age. However, it is apparent that these goals are not always achieved.

Data from the British Health Foundation shows that a large proportion of the population do not achieve the physical activity guidelines. Many health benefits are associated with physical exercise, for example exercise develops healthy bones, muscles, and joints, besides strengthening the heart and lungs, while it also refines coordination and movement control, in addition to the social aspects of exercise such as being outdoors, confidence, social interaction and integration. While a sedentary lifestyle is associated with an increased risk of developing heart disease, diabetes, stroke or obesity.

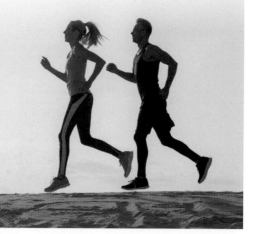

Age	Recommendation	Percentage meeting recommendation	
Children		**Male**	**Female**
2-4 years	At least 180 minutes (3 hours), spread throughout the day	9%	10%
5-10 years	At least 60 minutes and up to several hours every day	25%	20%
11-15 years	At least 60 minutes and up to several hours every day	17%	11%
Adults		**Male**	**Female**
19-64 years	Over one week, activity should add up to at least 150 minutes (2½ hours) of moderate intensity activity	67%	55%
65+ years	Over one week, activity should add up to at least 150 minutes (2½ hours) of moderate intensity activity	Age 65 – 74 58% Age 75+ 36%	Age 65 – 74 52% Age 75+ 18%

British Heart Foundation (2015) Physical Activity Statistics 2015.

Smoking

Smoking and vaping are popular social and stress relief activities. Yet it is widely published that smoking is highly associated with serious long term health conditions, such as heart disease, chronic obstructive pulmonary disease, stroke, lung disease and diabetes. While early indicators suggest that vaping may be associated with coronary heart disease, chronic obstructive pulmonary disease, and other lung diseases. Although these activities are often used as coping strategies, they can often mask a further health condition, which may include mental health, anxiety and depression. The main detrimental effect of smoking is the production of free radicals which attack tissues and exert oxidative damage. This tissue damage can occur anywhere in the body and can be especially serious if it occurs in the brain or other major organs whereby a health condition could develop. It is wise to reduce the number of cigarettes smoked with the aim to give up. There are several useful 'Stop Smoking Service' programmes available at local GP surgeries.

Alcohol

While an occasional glass of wine is reflective of the Mediterranean diet, a gradual increase in alcohol consumption to beyond 14 units each week is not ideal. As a largely preventable cause of death, excessive drinking of alcohol has been associated with at least 60 health conditions which include liver disease, an inflamed pancreas, gastrointestinal problems, immune disruption, brain damage which may be characterised by blurred vision, memory lapses and slowed reaction time, besides nutrient deficiencies, osteoporosis, and heart disease. Due to the way the liver detoxifies alcohol, a small amount several times each week is far less damaging than a large amount once a week. The Alcohol Change UK website offers a unit calculator which then notifies you of the number of units and calories consumed in alcohol each week.

Stress

Stress is important for motivation, but it is crucial that once the event is over, that stress levels return to a lowered level. However, in the modern, fast paced, high-pressured lifestyles psychological and physical stress can be elevated for a long duration. In response to stress several changes occur in the body so that we can cope. These include increased blood pressure and heart rate, the down regulation of immunity and reproductive organs plus the temporary cessation of non-essential functions such as digestion and motility besides the liberation of fatty acids into the blood stream and calorie dense food seeking behaviours - think about times when you might crave something sweet or fat laden like fast food. Although these functions aim to preserve life, they can contribute as risk factors to heart disease, elevated blood pressure, muscle damage, infertility, gastrointestinal upset, constipation or diarrhoea and infections when they become long term adaptations.

Social connections

Social connections create a sense of belonging which is highly important for human beings. Our ancestry revolved around being part of a tribe, which ensured regular feeding, communally raising children and safety, subsequently, to be outcast meant certain death. These characteristics are deeply imbedded and although we no longer dwell as tribes, loneliness and isolation can be common and physically damaging. Thus, highlighting the need for connection, socialisation, and companionship. Lack thereof has been associated with increased blood pressure, heart disease, obesity, a weak immune system, anxiety and depression, besides cognitive decline, dementia, and death.

Why is lifestyle so important?

All aspects of lifestyle have a huge impact on quality of life and health. Lifestyle encompasses family and social connections, exercise, and a decreased overall toxin load through not smoking and minimal alcohol consumption alongside a balanced diet. Quite the juggling act, but incredibly important for supporting health and minimising the risk of developing not only a single long term health condition but multiple conditions. It can be useful to assess your current lifestyle to see exactly what impact factors such as work environments, technology or home life has on your lifestyle decisions. Can these inputs be manipulated so that your lifestyle is enhanced and healthy for 80% of the time?

The work environment

Work routine and time spent commuting to and from work can take up a huge proportion of the day, meaning that if the work environment is not conducive to the healthful decisions this can have a huge impact. For instance, there may be difficulties accessing healthful foods, yet chocolates, cakes and biscuits are freely available. Social research shows that having these items hidden from sight and out of reach can reduce consumption. Plus, access to fruits, vegetables and nuts and seeds can support healthful choices in the workplace.

Eating is a routine

Fasting, shift work, and last-minute changes to your daily routine can disrupt eating patterns. However, it can be important to be prepared. This may be some fruit or nuts to snack on should a meal be delayed. The crucial aspect of eating patterns is not necessarily the time that you eat but managing hunger queues and never becoming ravenous. The overall caloric intake and allowing for a 12-hour overnight fast has been shown to be highly beneficial in terms of blood glucose values, body mass and digestive health. For example, if an evening meal is eaten at 8pm, and so breakfast should not be consumed until at least 8am the following day.

Technology - a tool or hindrance?

The boon of technology is the plethora of useful apps that track everything from activity to calorie intake. These can be used to track and maintain routine. However, technology can become a hindrance when perspective is lost. This may be via unachievable desires motivated by social media, or the expectation to achieve calorie intake and activity goals 100% of the time. A small relaxation of expectations to an 80% success rate is achievable and allows for slight, guilt free deviations which do not signal a complete failure.

Travel disruption

Regular travel, whether it is work based or for leisure is pleasurable, but it can mess up routines. You can be crossing time zones, find it difficult to add in a leisure activity, eat unfamiliar foods, add in a few extra units of alcohol, and even struggle to find the time to chat with your family and friends. These disruptions can make it difficult to stick to a healthy lifestyle and dietary pattern. It can be useful to be prepared, look up the restaurant menu, is there a gym or a park near your accommodation where you can exercise. Planning a solution can make the activity pleasurable and create a feeling of maintaining control over your choices.

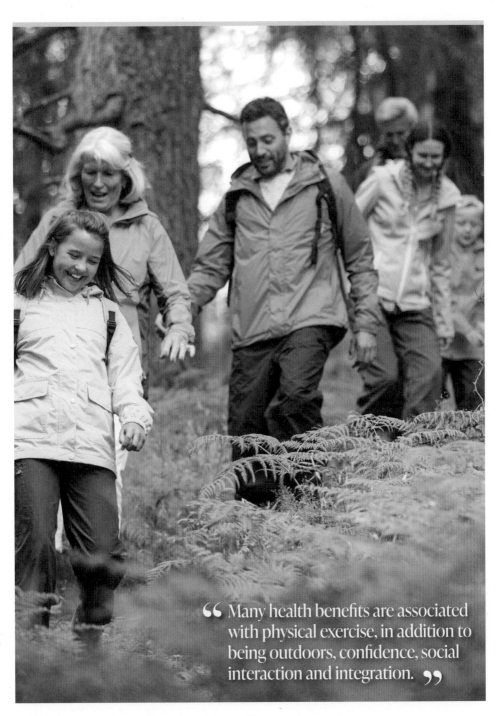

> **Many health benefits are associated with physical exercise, in addition to being outdoors, confidence, social interaction and integration.**

Food hide and seek

Food deserts are a phenomenon of a fast-food outlet influenced society. Commonly found in low socioeconomic suburban areas where there is an abundance of fast-food outlets and small shops that vend highly processed foods but limited access to fresh produce. This makes access to wholefoods extremely difficult, thus following a varied and balanced diet is near impossible. Similarly, work location may mean that the only source of food is a nearby petrol station and so this emphasises the need to prepare healthful foods and to make food preparation a habit.

Home life obstacles

Ferrying children to after school clubs, taking the dog to the vets and collecting family members from the train station soon eats into time and energy. Home life can be hectic and motivation to cook after a busy day may wane. In addition, there is less time available for the planning, shopping for and preparation of healthy meals, lunches and breakfasts.

66 **In areas with a high proportion of people aged over 100, the diet consists of mainly plant based meals** 99

Sedentary

A reduction in activity commonly occurs in people with disease, long term health conditions, in the elderly and certain people with obesity. These individuals may face several barriers to healthy food choices, that include a reliance on food services such as meals on wheels, carers, healthcare professionals, and their mobility. In inactive people there can be some weight loss, but it is often primarily muscle wasting and so the individual will experience a reduction in their caloric requirements.

However, in able bodied individuals there are several health campaigns to promote regular exercise and a healthy lifestyle such as 'Couch to 5K'.

Changes to lifestyle play a huge role in health outcomes. Several studies have investigated those populations that have a high proportion of centenarians (people aged over 100) to gain an understanding of what factors play a role into healthful longevity. Blue Zones is such an organisation that publishes research and helps communities to promote health and longevity.

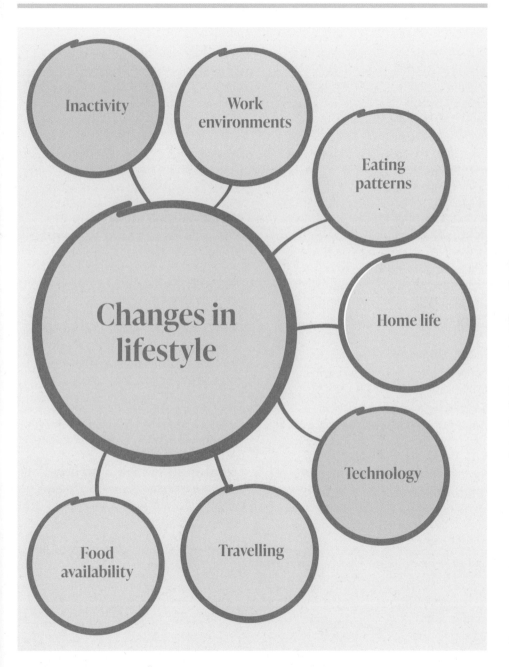

There are many elements that can impact a healthy lifestyle.

The habits of centenarians

Blue Zones classify the locations around the world that have the highest density of centenarians. They are shown to have nine factors in common that are considered to be responsible for longer, healthier, and happier lives.

1. **Move naturally**
   Exercise is via environmental design. Those living in Blue Zones do not 'keep fit' they grow gardens, travel by foot or bicycle and use manual tools for house and garden work.

2. **Purpose**
   Knowing your sense of purpose is worth up to seven extra years of life.

3. **Downshift**
   Adopt a lifestyle that has a low level of stress plus practice gratitude or meditate.
   Making time for an afternoon nap can be refreshing.

4. **80% rule**
   Stop eating when you are 80% full.

5. **Plant slant**
   Eat meals that are mostly plant based

6. **Wine at 5**
   A small daily glass of wine is a commonality.

7. **Right tribe**
   Developing groups of five friends that show up for each other.

8. **Loved ones**
   Families come first and generally several generations will live close by.

9. **Belonging**
   Participation in a community is vital whether it is faith based or other, such as sport, discussion or social groups.

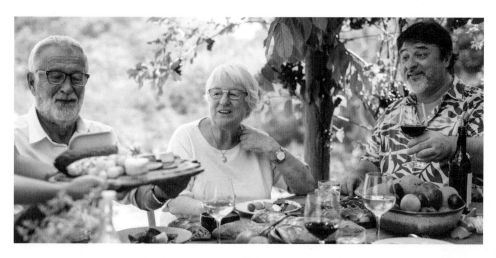

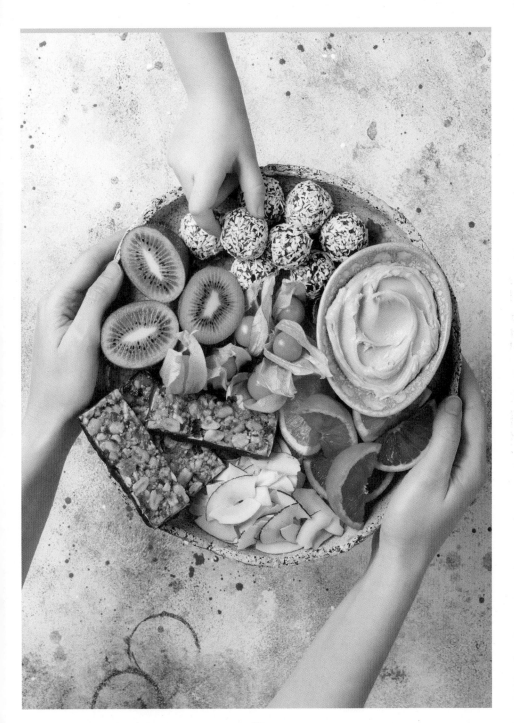

Convenient Swaps

Although the perception of convenience foods is that they are the perfect solution for the time poor individual, knowledge on their nutrient provision is lacking. And so, convenience foods remain popular, however simple swaps and alternatives are just as quick and easy but also provide a whole load of nutrition.

90 days to change your life

It's never too late to take the right path, just 90 days of a wholefood regimen can make a significant difference to your biomarkers and change your habits ongoing.

Convenience	Simple Swap
Ready meal	Slow cooker chickpea and lentil pilaf or a meat joint with veggies and herbs.
Pizza	Omelette base 'pizza'
Breakfast bars	Homemade oat bars
Prepack sandwich	Couscous salad
Sweets	Fruit, especially frozen grapes and frozen berries
Biscuits	A handful of raw walnuts and/or almonds

Ready meal swap

A slow cooker can transform food preparation. It simply requires adding the food to the cooker plus enough water so that it does not dry out and switch on for 4-6 hours depending on the ingredients.

A chickpea and lentil pilaf takes just ten minutes to prepare and four hours on low or medium setting. Remember to add three times the volume of stock to the dried chickpeas, lentils and rice. Throw in a chopped onion, garlic and kale or cabbage, plus season with oregano, cumin, turmeric and chili powder. While a meat joint can be packed in with root vegetables and covered in water to cook on the medium setting for six hours. And hey presto, your meal is ready as you walk through the door.

Pizza swap

Pizza is the perfect comfort food, but often it is laden in empty calories from processed oils and topped with preformed meats.

The omelette pizza takes no more than ten minutes to prepare and cook. The base requires 2-3 eggs whisked with a splash of milk and some herbs then cooked in a large frying pan. Once the base is cooked through cover in tomato slices, wilted and squeezed dry spinach, plus toppings, such as pineapple, fresh vegetables, olives, or tofu, then sprinkle with grated mozzarella. Cover and cook until the cheese is melted.

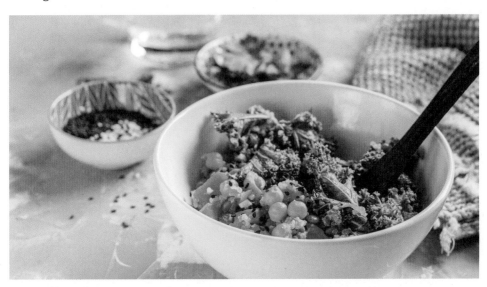

Break the fast swap

Breakfast bars are easy to go to, but surprisingly they are full of salt and sugar, so in actual fact you will be hungry an hour or so later. However, if you commit 30 minutes at the weekend to make your own you will have 12 bars that sustain your hunger and nourish your body after you break the overnight fast.

Soak 2 tablespoons of chia and flaxseeds in 6 tablespoons of water for at least 10 minutes, meanwhile, chop 6 medjool dates and mash 2 bananas together. Add 400g of oats to the dates and bananas, mix then add the chia and flaxseeds and mix again thoroughly, spice with cinnamon or mixed spices. You may need to add more water until the mixture becomes sticky then put it into a baking tray, slice into 12 bars and bake for 10-15 minutes at 160C. This recipe can be altered by using milk or milk alternatives instead of water and a selection of dried fruits instead of dates.

Pre-pack swap

Pre-packaged sandwiches are a staple for many time-strapped employees. But how many would say they truly enjoy that sandwich? Generally soggy and devoid of fresh vegetables or salad but loaded with mayo and other salty 'delights'. They spike blood glucose, evade satiety and may contribute to the mid-afternoon slump.

Couscous is a quick-to-cook grain, just 5 minutes soaking in boiling water and the grains are good to go. Add torn lettuce or leaves, cucumber, tomatoes, olives and feta, you can top it with a boiled egg or some oily fish and season with garam masala and coriander leaf.

Sweet swap

A packet of sweets can be consumed far quicker than expected, with no effect on hunger levels. Try freezing grapes and berries and eating those instead of sweets. The combination of the natural sweetness and the frozen state makes them taste like sweets but without the sugar, colourants artificial flavours and preservatives.

Take the biscuit (swap)

When all you want is the crunch factor, biscuits often fulfil that urge. However, so do raw nuts, especially walnuts and almonds. In fact, any nut will do, and they soon quell the crunch craving. An extension to this swap is to cut celery and carrots into sticks and dip them into one tablespoon of nut butter.

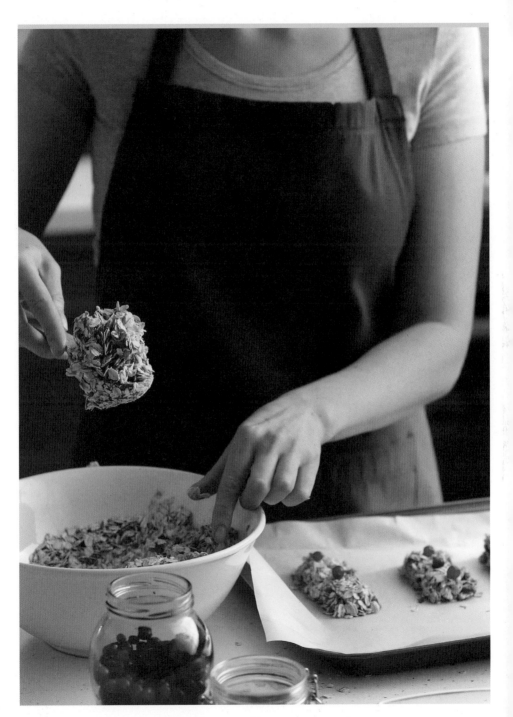

Conclusion

There is a clearly a very obvious relationship between the Western diet and the onset and progression of serious long term health conditions, but throughout this book, we've seen there are simple steps that can be taken, via dietary and lifestyle changes, to stall or even reverse poor health and set you on the wellness path.

We have discussed the importance of including a wide variety of "rainbow" foods and their subsequent nutrients in the diet to support life phases, specific symptoms, and prescription medication.

A careful consideration of the pressures, responsibilities, activities, time allocated to exercise, and relaxation will help you to assess whether your diet and lifestyle contributes to your health goals, provides the necessary nutrition and what specific supplementation would be wise. Further support to help you to assess your personalised regime can be found in your local health food store, where they'll also be pleased to chat through any specific wellbeing concerns you have.

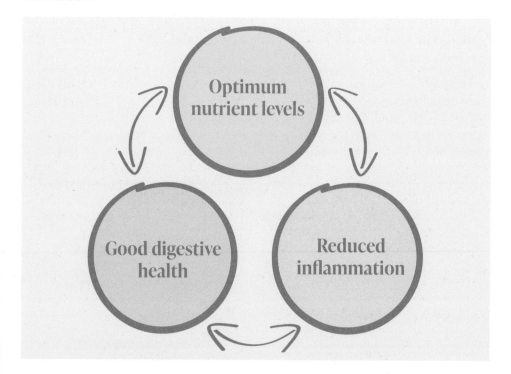

The nutrition trinity to support your health

> Three key elements support abundant health: nourishment, inflammation and digestion.

1. Optimum nutrient levels

Earlier sections have shown that modern living has added additional nutritional requirements and the trend for processed, quick foods doesn't meet these requirements. They may even introduce the risk of oxidative damage and DNA damage through compounds such as trans-fats. A wide variety of rainbow-coloured wholefoods will help to achieve a nutrient dense diet.

A daily multivitamin can help to provide all the essential nutrients necessary for health, especially when we're under pressure and eating on the run. Several population groups are at greater risk of being under-nourished: the elderly, during pregnancy and lactation, those following a restricted diet (calorie-controlled weight loss, vegetarians and vegans), smokers, drinkers, athletes, those with malabsorption conditions and those taking medications that are known to deplete certain nutrients. Choose multivitamin supplements that are tailored to your personal needs, are effective, ethical and pure, never-GMO and free from excipients.

2. Minimising long term inflammation

Quite often hidden inside the body.

It is clear that inflammation plays a beneficial role in the prevention and management of infections, however, the risk is when inflammation becomes out of control and spreads throughout the body. Unmanaged chronic inflammation can be damaging and trigger oxidative damage which puts huge demands on energy provision to maintain, specifically a demand that cannot be met over a long duration. This then puts the body at further risk of developing secondary and tertiary health conditions.

As well as their anti-inflammatory properties, we've seen that fats are necessary for hormonal health, energy, brain and skin health. Evidence shows that a diet balanced in omega-6 and omega-3 essential fatty acids may have the capacity to prevent and stall the progression of many long-term health conditions. For many, supplemental nutritional oils may be considered. omega-3 essential fatty acids rich options include organic fish oils, algae and flaxseed oil. Ideally, choose an organic, high quality, pure nutritional oil, without additives.

3. Maximising digestive health

The gastrointestinal tract is often considered the source of all health and all illness.

It is considered that the gut microbiome is so dynamic that every single meal affects the diversity and function. Optimising the microbiome takes several factors, the introduction of beneficial bacteria, sufficient dietary resistant fibres and a low stress lifestyle. We now understand that supplements combining probiotics and prebiotics, known as synbiotics, can be used to support general health and improve specific conditions.

Health is individual, it can be influenced by genetics, however the biggest influences are diet, lifestyle and environmental exposures. By following a predominantly wholefood diet with gentle exercise and a nutritional programme of appropriate supplements including a targeted multivitamin, a probiotic and a nutritional oil, you are giving yourself the best possible chance to preserve health. By following this plan for 90 days, you'll develop daily habits that will last you a lifetime.

Dietary and lifestyle change will vary dependant on your current health situation, there will be difficult and easy aspects, but purely starting is the biggest challenge you will encounter.

Your body will thank you, and your friends and family will look on in awe – maybe your joyful transformation will influence them to consider whether they are living their best lives.

Remember though, perfection is a non-entity, the ideal lifestyle involves balance. Making healthy choices 80% of the time allows for 20% flexibility, so be kind to yourself and when you choose a pizza or a piece of cake, enjoy it, mindful that your next meal will be wholefoods.

Wishing you a life filled with abundant health and happiness.

Jenny x.

Why Visit Health Stores

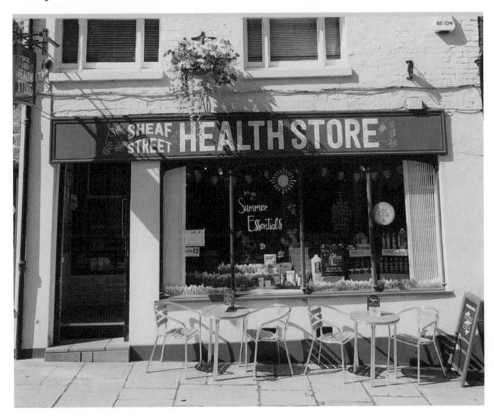

Choosing the right supplement programme for your personal needs can be confusing. Allow the staff at your local specialist health store to take you through the vitamin maze, where trained and knowledgeable advisors are on hand to develop the ideal programme of nutritional supplements just for you.

Where else would someone take you by the hand, offer a shoulder to cry on, a listening ear, a knowledgeable mind and kind heart?

If you have a particular health condition or concern, please first visit a health professional (a GP or a qualified practitioner) to ensure you have the correct diagnosis. Often with chronic health conditions, the health food store will give excellent advice for dietary and lifestyle modifications, a supplement programme and possibly assistance from topical products.

References and Further Resources

Bienz, D., 2003. Adequate dosing of micronutrients for different age groups in the life cycle. Food and Nutrition Bulletin, 24(3):S7-S15.

Bourre JM. Effects of nutrients (in food) on the structure and function of the nervous system: update on dietary requirements for brain. Part 1: micronutrients. J Nutr Health Aging. 2006 Sep-Oct;10(5):377-85.

British Nutrition Foundation. 2021. An active lifestyle. Pages 1-8. [Online] Accessed: https://www.nutrition.org.uk/healthyliving/an-active-lifestyle/how-much-physical-activity-do-i-need.html?limitstart=0 24 August 2021.

British Nutrition Foundation. 2016. Nutrition Requirements. [Online] Accessed: https://www.nutrition.org.uk/attachments/article/234/Nutrition%20Requirements_Revised%20Oct%202016.pdf 27 August 2021.

British Heart Foundation (2015) Physical Activity Statistics 2015.

Broderick, NA. 2015. A common origin for Immunity and Digestion. Front Immunol. 6:72.

Buettner, D., Power 9: Reverse Engineering Longevity. Blue Zones. [Online] Accessed: https://www.bluezones.com/2016/11/power-9/ 24 August 2021.

Calton, J.B. Prevalence of micronutrient deficiency in popular diet plans. J Int Soc Sports Nutr 7, 24 (2010).

Carabotti, M., et al. 2015. The gut-brain axis: interactions between enteric microbiota, central and enteric nervous systems. Ann Gastroenterol. 28(2):203-9.

Cordain et al. 2005. Origins and evolution of the Western diet: Health implications for the 21st century. American Journal of Clinical Nutrition; 81:341-54.

Department of Health (2012). Long-term conditions compendium of information: 3rd edition.

Dimidi, E. et al. 2019. Fermented foods: Definitions and characteristics, impact on the gut microbiota and effects on gastrointestinal health and disease. Nutrients. 11(8): 1806.

Eby GA, Eby KL. Rapid recovery from major depression using magnesium treatment. Med Hypotheses. 2006;67(2):362-70.

Freeman, K., Ryan, R., Parsons, N. et al. The incidence and prevalence of inflammatory bowel disease in UK primary care: a retrospective cohort study of the IQVIA Medical Research Database. BMC Gastroenterol 21, 139 (2021).

Freeman MP, Hibbeln JR, Silver M, Hirschberg AM, Wang B, Yule AM, Petrillo LF, Pascuillo E, Economou NI, Joffe H, Cohen LS. omega-3 fatty acids for major depressive disorder associated with the menopausal transition: a preliminary open trial. Menopause. 2011 Mar;18(3):279-84.

Gillespie, S., van den Bold, M., Agriculture, Food Systems, and Nutrition: Meeting the Challenge. Global Challenges 2017, 1, 1600002.

Kantar 2019. 38% of adults say they are trying to lose weight. [Online] Accessed: https://www.kantar.com/uki/inspiration/consumer/38-percent-of-uk-adults-say-they-are-trying-to-lose-weight 25 August 2021.

Kantar https://www.kantar.com/uki/inspiration/consumer/38-percent-of-uk-adults-say-they-are-trying-to-lose-weight

Kechagia, A., et al. 2013. Health benefits of probiotics: A review. ISRN Nutr.2013:481651.

Kiens, CL., et al. 2013. Substituting dietary monounsaturated fat for saturated fat is associated with increased daily physical activity and resting energy expenditure and with changes in mood. Am J Clin Nutr. 98(2):511.

Kings College (2018) From one to many: Exploring people's progression to multiple long-term conditions in an urban environment. Guy's & St Thomas' Charity. 1(1):1-55.

Levenson CW. Zinc: the new antidepressant? Nutr Rev. 2006 Jan;64(1):39-42.

Lukaski HC. Vitamin and mineral status: effects on physical performance. Nutrition. 2004 Jul-Aug;20(7-8):632-44.

Marklund, M., 2019. Biomarkers of dietary omega-6 fatty acids and incident cardiovascular disease and mortality. Circulation. 139(21):2422-36.

Mozaffarian D, Rosenberg I, Uauy R. History of modern nutrition science—implications for current research, dietary guidelines, and food policy BMJ 2018; 361 :k2392

Overton, M., 2011. Agricultural Revolution in England 1500 – 1850. [Online] Accessed: http://www.bbc.co.uk/history/british/empire_seapower/agricultural_revolution_01.shtml 25 August 2021.

Pahwa R, Goyal A, Bansal P, et al. Chronic Inflammation. [Updated 2020 Nov 20]. In: StatPearls [Internet]. Treasure Island (FL): StatPearls Publishing; 2021 Jan-.

Pes, G., et al. 2011. Lifestyle and nutrition related to male longevity in Sardinia: An ecological study. Nutrition Metabolism and Cardiovascular Diseases, xx:1-8.

Public Health England. 2020. Research and analysis: Prescribed medicines review summary. [Online] Accessed: https://www.gov.uk/government/publications/prescribed-medicines-review-report/prescribed-medicines-review-summary#:~:text=PHE%20's%20analysis%20shows%20that,the%20review%20%5Bfootnote%201%5D. 26 August 2021.

Ritz P, Elia M. The effect of inactivity on dietary intake and energy homeostasis. Proc Nutr Soc. 1999 Feb;58(1):115-22.

Simopoulos AP. The importance of the ratio of omega-6/ omega-3 essential fatty acids. Biomed Pharmacother. 2002 Oct;56(8):365-79.

Singer, S. 2018. Health Effects of Social Isolation and Loneliness. Journal of Aging Life Care, Spr:4-8.

Tardivo AP, Nahas-Neto J, Orsatti CL, Dias FB, Poloni PF, Schmitt EB, Nahas EA. Effects of omega-3 on metabolic markers in postmenopausal women with metabolic syndrome. Climacteric. 2015 Apr;18(2):290-8.

Thomas, D,. 2003. A study on the mineral depletion of the foods available to us as a nation over the period 1940 to 1991. Nutrition and Health Journal. 17(2):85-115.

Tuomisto, H., Effects of environmental change on agriculture, nutrition and health: A framework with a focus on fruits and vegetables. Version 2. Wellcome Open Res. 2017; 2: 21.

Unwin D, Khalid AA, Unwin J, et al. Insights from a general practice service evaluation supporting a lower carbohydrate diet in patients with type 2 diabetes mellitus and prediabetes: a secondary analysis of routine clinic data including HbA1c, weight and prescribing over 6 years

BMJ Nutrition, Prevention & Health 2020;3.

Vangay, P., et al. 2018. US immigration westernizes the human gut microbiome. Cell. 175(4):962-72.

Zajicek, G. 1994. The normal and the pathological; Editorial. The Cancer Journal. 7(2):48-9.

Zinocker, MK, and Lindseth, IA., 2018. The Western diet-microbiome-host interaction and its role in metabolic disease. Nutrients. 10(3):365.

Further Resources

The Viridian Nutrition range is available from carefully selected health food stores and specialist health counters worldwide.

Health food stores offer expertise, range and care.

Reading materials available at health stores:
- Allergies
- Black Seed, a 3000 Year Old Secret
- Cardiovascular Health
- Children's Health
- Clear Skin
- Digestive Health
- Energy & Vitality
- Fertility and Pregnancy
- Joint Health & Flexibility
- Magnesium
- Nutritional Balance for a Vegan Diet
- Nutrition For Brain Health
- Organic Health
- Probiotics & Prebiotics
- Scandinavian Rainbow Trout Oil
- Skin, Hair & Nails
- Stress, Sleep & Mood
- The Sunshine Vitamin
- Vitamin C
- Winter Wellness
- Women's Health
- 60 Day Clear Skin Programme
- The 7 Day Sugar Detox Plan

To find your nearest independent health store visit:
findahealthstore.com

Ethical vitamins
with an organic heart

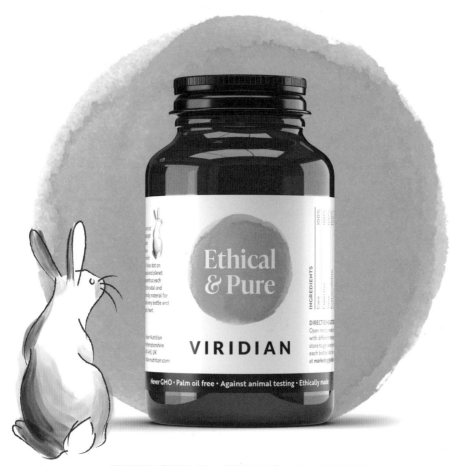

EFFECTIVE, ETHICAL, PURE

Recommended with confidence by experts at independent health stores

VIRIDIAN